The Expansion of Consciousness

ALSO BY RALPH METZNER

Sacred Vine of Spirits – Ayahuasca (2006; Editor)

Sacred Mushroom of Visions – Teonanácatl (2005; Editor)

Green Psychology: Transforming our Relationship to the Earth (1999)

The Unfolding Self: Varieties of Transformative Experience (1998)

The Well of Remembrance: Earth Wisdom Myths of Northern Europe (1994)

Through the Gateway of the Heart: Accounts of Experiences with MDMA and other Empathogenic Substances (1985; Editor)

Know Your Type: Maps of Identity (1979)

Maps of Consciousness: I Ching, Tantra, Tarot, Alchemy, Astrology, Actualism (1971)

The Ecstatic Adventure (1968; Editor)

The Psychedelic Experience: A Manual Based on the Tibetan Book of the Dead (1964; co-authored with Timothy Leary and Richard Alpert)

THE

EXPANSION OF CONSCIOUSNESS

by
Ralph Metzner

I The Quest for the Alchemical Philosopher's Stone

II Expansions of Collective Consciousness
– A Brief History Since the End of WWII

Green Earth Foundation
& REGENT PRESS

ISBN 13: 978-1-58790-147-8
ISBN 10: 1-58790-147-1
Library of Congress Control Number: 2007943347

Published by
REGENT PRESS
www.regentpress.net
for
GREEN EARTH FOUNDATION
www.greenearthfound.org

Manufactured in the U.S.A.
REGENT PRESS
2747 Regent Street
Berkeley, CA 94705
e-mail: regentpress@mindspring..com

Printed on 30% post-consumer recycled fiber,
archival [acid free] paper

Acknowledgements

Both of these essays were first written as lectures for the international symposium in Basel, Switzerland, on the occasion of Albert Hofmann's 100th birthday, January 2006. I am grateful to Dieter Hagenbach, Lucius Werthmüller and Michael Gasser of the Gaia Media Stiftung, the organizers, for their invitation to participate in this superbly organized conference; to Roger Liggenstorfer of the Nachtschatten Verlag in Solothurn, publisher of the symposium volume *Albert Hofmann und die Entdeckung des LSD,* which included the Alchemy essay; and to Mathias Broeckers, his co-editor on that volume, who did the German translation of both essays. Many thanks also to Roger for inviting the publication of a separate booklet that would incorporate these two essays; and to Mathias, Berlin journalist and author, for stimulating conversation on the ideas of the second essay.

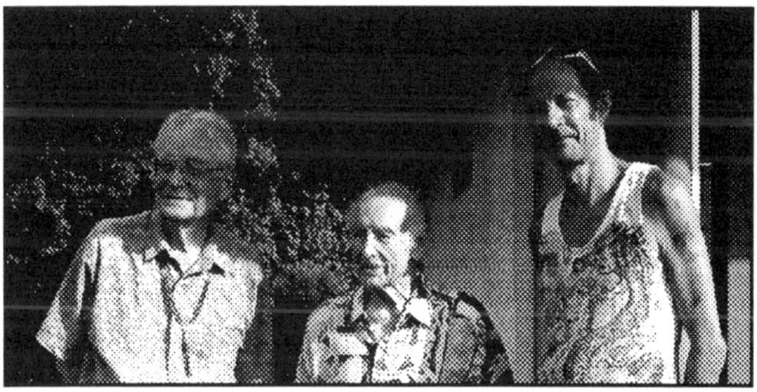

Ralph Metzner, Albert Hofmann, Roger Liggenstorfer, Rittimatte, June 2006

I have benefitted from several discussants of these essays, for which I am deeply grateful. Michael Flanagin, long-term student of C.G. Jung's work, gave me detailed and subtle comments on the first essay, which clarified my understanding of Jung's concept of the "transcendent function." Micah and Paul, practical lab alchemists of the Al-Kemi company, producers of Spagyric medicinal essences, supported me in my view of the intimate interdependence of the material and psychic aspects of alchemical work.

I was also fortunate to be able to discuss the ideas of the second essay, on the transformations of collective consciousness, with long-term friends and colleagues Stanislav Grof and Richard Tarnas. The latter's ground-breaking book, *Cosmos and Psyche,* on the archetypal planetary patterns of historical transformation, appeared in the Spring of 2006. While I wrote my essay originally using a different transformative model, I was thrilled to find, in his writings, confirmations and extensions of the dynamics of societal change that I was seeing. Readers, who wish to explore these in greater depth and detail, will find *Cosmos and Psyche* a treasure-house of insight and erudition.

I am further grateful to my assistant Cynthia Smith, for her skillful work on designing the layout of the book, and preparing it for publication.

The present volume is the first in a series of six booklets of my writings, under the general title of *THE ECOLOGY OF CONSCIOUSNESS*, being published by the Green Earth Foundation (see back of the book for details). I am deeply grateful to the following individuals for their financial support for this venture: Robert J. Barnhart, John Buchanan, Uwe and Cathy Doerken, Elizabeth Gordon, Michael Kahn, George Kapnas, Bill and Lynne Twist and Richard M. Wolfe.

Contents

The Quest for the Alchemical Philosophers Stone[1]

Alchemy, descended from shamanism, is the ancient art and science of elemental transformation. The historian of religion Mircea Eliade in his book *The Forge and the Crucible,* posited that alchemy grew historically out of the work of shamanic miners, smiths and metallurgists (Eliade, 1962). They were the masters of fire, who knew how to extract metals (like copper, tin, iron, gold, silver) from stone, blend them into alloys such as bronze, and make tools (like adz, hammer, plow), weapons (like spear, sword, dagger, shield) and ornaments (like necklace, bracelet, crown, ring). In the archaic and classical period the knowledge of metal-working, because of its obvious connection to power and wealth, was preserved in secrecy and handed down in craft-guilds from master to student. Such technical knowledge was regarded as *magical* by ordinary people, because it seemed to involve inexplicable mastery of natural forces. The crafts of masonry, which uses mineral stones in building, and medicine, which uses mineral and botanical extracts in healing (as well as metal tools in surgery), were parallel and associated secret societies. All three movements developed an esoteric or inner component, concerned with practices of psychic and spiritual self-transformation.

A popular misconception is that alchemy was solely and futilely concerned with the transmutation of base metals to gold. In actuality, it is clear from alchemical writings that the main focus of most alchemical practitioners was healing and what we would nowadays call psychotherapy: the *transmutation of the physical and psychic condition of the human being – starting with oneself.* The worldview of the archaic and classical eras was *holistic* – the physical, psychic, spiritual and cosmic dimensions of life were seen in their wholeness, not as separate fields. As such, alchemy can be considered a specialized extension of the shamanic traditions of healing and transformation dating from the Old Stone Age. Shamans in surviving indigenous societies also have specialized knowledge of plants and mineral substances, including crystals, and secret initiatory knowledge of the spiritual dimensions. They negotiate with the normally inaccessible spirits of nature and the ancestors on behalf of their clients.

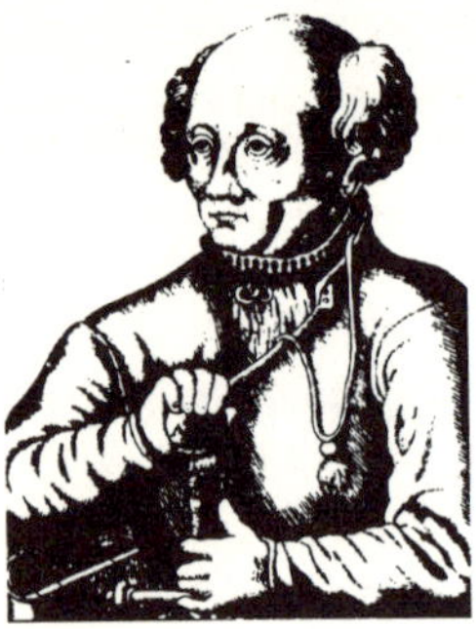

Paracelsus 1493-1541

Alchemists, like shamans, worked with *spirits*, in particular the spirits of the elements (air, fire, earth and water) and certain deities (Hephaestos for the Greeks, Vulcanus for the Romans) that were the guides and teachers of mining and blacksmithing. The great 16th century alchemical adept Paracelsus identified and named the spirits associated with the four elements: the air spirits were called *elves*, the water spirits *undines*, the earth spirits *gnomes*, and the fire spirits *salamanders.* In Germanic-Norse mythology, the spirits of stone, metal and fire were called the "black elves" *(Schwarzalben)* or dwarves. Their home world, called *Schwarzalfheim*, was underground, in the stones, rocks and mountains. Like the giants, who are the spirits of vast natural aggregates like mountain ranges, forests, rivers and storms, the dark elves were neither benevolent nor malevolent toward humans. They were said to have their own agenda, neutral in regard to human welfare and survival. But humans could communicate with them and learn from them, if one had the access codes, so to speak. One could say that those human beings who worked as miners and smiths, the makers of metal weapons, tools and ornaments, were in fact inspired and taught by these stone-spirits, these black elves.

The dwarves or black elves were highly respected for their knowledge and skills in tool and weapon making, but they were not the kinds of spirits with which one had friendly relations. As I have described in my book *The Well of Remembrance* (Metzner, 1994), the myths of Odin/Wotan, the knowledge-seeking god of shamans and warriors, tell of him wandering the worlds asking questions – of dwarves, as well as gods, goddesses, elves, giants and humans, and even the dead (which is *necromancy*). Other gods also, communicated and obtained knowledge from the dwarves. One of the poems of the *Eddas* relates a dialogue between the thunder god Thor and a very knowledgeable dwarf called *Allwiss,* the "All-knowing One," who is interested in marrying Thor's daughter. Wanting to test and discourage his daughter's suitor, Thor poses a series of more and more difficult linguistic puzzles, which the knowledgeable dwarf successfully answers, until he is overcome by the light of day.

I find the mythic image of the spirits of metal and stone suggestive, in view of the morally questionable though technically skillful nature of many of the technologies that modern science has loosed upon the world. We can see in this ancient mythic conception an understanding of the principle that the knowledge of natural forces and tools is morally neutral: it can be used for health and creativity, in the service of the divine and of life; but when used for personal aggrandizement, domination and enrichment at the expense of others, it becomes sorcery, black magic, the "dark side." Shamans, alchemists, doctors, wizards or witches, or modern scientists, who use their knowledge and power, and knowledge of the spirits of nature, to heal and serve others are contributing to the well-being of the community and society. Those who use their knowledge and power for the accumulation of wealth and personal power over others, serve only the individual or a select group – not the whole.

Paleolithic shamanism developed knowledge and methods of healing transformation, by accessing the hidden spiritual forces behind or within the phenomena of the world of nature around them. In the Egyptian and Greco-Roman civilizations alchemy developed as the extension and continuation of this Paleolithic practice and science – as empirically tested technologies of physico-psychic-spiritual transformation. In India, the transformative practices of shamans and alchemists developed into the psycho-spiritual practices of Yoga. Mircea Eliade, in his book *Yoga, Immortality and Freedom*, showed that yoga was crucially concerned with practices that liberate consciousness from the thrall of the material sense world – this was called the path of *mukti* – liberation (Eliade, 1969). Alchemical texts also exist in the Indian yogic healing tradition, known as Ayurveda, and are often concerned with the use of psychoactive and medicinal plant, fungal or mineral substances. A central concept of alchemical tantric yoga was *rasa* – which means something like "essence," "tincture," "feeling," and "taste." This strand of the yogic tradition was called *rasayana*, "the way of cultivating essence."

Alchemy is also known in Chinese Taoism, where it is an integral aspect of the Taoist preoccupations with longevity (called "immortality") and the yogic practices of recycling sexual energies for regeneration. It appears that in the Indian and Chinese traditions, the physical, psychic and spiritual aspects of the transformational work remained more or less connected, although sub-schools arose which focused on one or another aspect (e.g. *hatha yoga* on the physical, *bhakti yoga* on the emotional). In the West, the alchemical practices of human elemental transformation originated in Egypt, spread to the Hellenistic and Arabic lands during the classical era, and flourished well into medieval times in Christian Europe.

The word "alchemy," which is the root of the word "chemistry," comes from the Arabic *al-kimiya* – "the science of the black earth land." *Kam*, or *Kem*, "Black Earth," was the ancient Egyptian name for their land, referring to the very fertile black earth along the Nile after the seasonal floods. It was the land of the Black Goddess (Nut, Isis, or Hathor), who transmuted into the Black Madonna in Christian times. The name points to the Egyptian origin of alchemy. At its greatest flowering, the ancient Egyptian civilization, which may indeed have been founded by an even earlier Atlantean or even extra-terrestrial civilization, embodied a completely integrated scientific, spiritual and artistic worldview, a *sacred science*, to use the term of the renowned Egyptologist Schwaller de Lubicz (West, 1993; Sitchin, 1976).

In the Hellenistic period, the god *Hermes*, who was *Thoth* or *Djehuti* to the Egyptians, and *Mercurius* to the Romans, emerged as the main deity or spirit guide of the alchemical work of transformation. Thoth was the scientist, scribe and record keeper among the gods. Hermes/Mercury was the divine messenger, carrying knowledge between the divine and human worlds – and thus the *practice of divination*. Mercury the metal, also called *quicksilver*, because of its highly mobile, fluid characteristics, became symbolically associated with the mind or awareness. Like quicksilver, the mind can slip and slide to strange elusive places, but it can also shine with sparkling brilliance. In addition to Hermes the god, there was also a legendary, very advanced human spiritual teacher, called *Hermes Trismegistos* ("Three-fold Great Hermes"). The appellation "Three-fold Great," refers perhaps to the three phases of manifestation of this divine being – as youth, as man and as old man, analogous to the mythic image of the Triple Goddess as maiden, mother and crone.

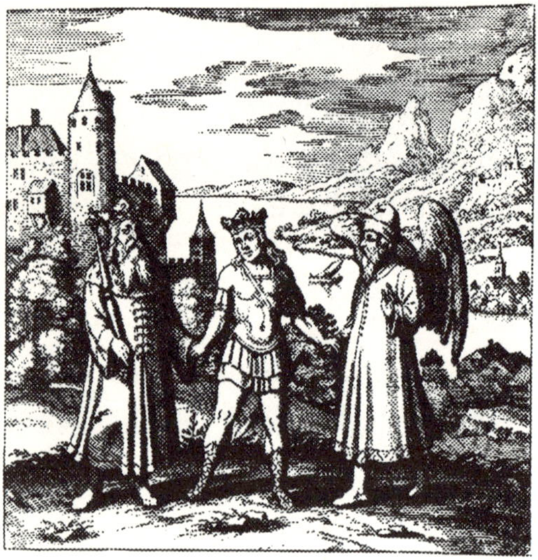

Three-fold Hermes
(from alchemical text by Lambsprinck, 1625)

This Hermes the Teacher-Adept founded a school of secret knowledge of self-transformation practices, that formed the core of European alchemy, which became known as the *Hermetic tradition.* Whereas one strand of this knowledge stream concerned itself with the transformation of physical matter, the making of tools, medicines and instruments, the esoteric, mystical core of it were the practices of psychospiritual self-transformation. The most important of the material tools, including plant or fungal or mineral tinctures, as well as metallic instruments, were those that contributed to the practices of consciousness transformation. The secrecy in this tradition was so profound that the term "hermetically sealed" is still a symbolic expression of absolute secrecy. The teachings of the school were not secret arbitrarily or for reasons of power and control, as is sometimes assumed. Rather, they were secret for the same reason that esoteric yogic and shamanic practices are kept secret – because misuse of the knowledge by those motivated by greed or power could have harmful consequences. Later, during the European Middle Ages, because of the persecutory dominance of the Catholic Church, such practices, like the practices of shamanic witchcraft, were shrouded in secrecy because of the very real danger of the Inquisition. Texts were written and illustrated, but in a symbolic code, known only to initiated students, and copied and passed on. The keys to the code were largely lost in the course of time, and the texts became increasingly garbled and incomprehensible.

Under the pressure of the persecutory ideological zeal of the Catholic Church over several centuries, the Hermetic tradition in Europe basically split into two strands during the time of the beginnings of the materialist science paradigm (16th & 17th centuries): one strand became what we call "chemistry" in modern times the precise quantitative, experimental investigations into transformation processes at the material level, but with no consideration given to the possible relationship of the material processes to the world of Spirit and higher forms of consciousness and knowledge. This other part of the tradition split off and went underground, became "occult" ("hidden"), as we say. A similar schism happened to the ancient holistic science of astrology, with one strand splitting off as scientific astronomy, and the other being relegated to the cultural underground as "superstition." It's interesting to recall that two of the founding giants of the scientific worldview – Isaac Newton and Johannes Kepler – were themselves deep students of these secret esoteric sciences. Newton spent 17

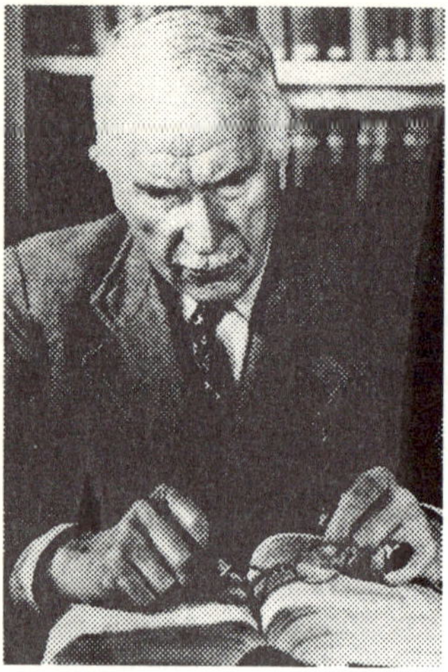

Carl Gustav Jung 1875-1961

years investigating alchemical texts and performing alchemical experiments in his laboratory, before going on to formulate the laws of motion for which he became famous. Kepler wrote major contributions to astrological thought, did occasional horoscopes for rulers and princes, and pursued his research into the orbital paths of the planets in the belief that he was uncovering the basic "harmonies of the cosmos" (which became the title of his major work – *Harmonices Mundi*).

It remained to C.G. Jung and his followers, in the 20th century, to recover the lost language of alchemy and re-interpret it as referring to psychospiritual transformation using symbolic and imaginal processes. Four of the twenty or so volumes of Jung's *Collected Works* are essentially alchemical texts: *Psychology and Alchemy, Alchemical Studies, Aion* and *Mysterium Coniunctionis.* In his profound scholarly studies of alchemical writings, Jung interprets the *opus* or "work" of alchemy as being the individuation process – the individual's moving toward wholeness. The alchemical vessel, called *athanor*, in which these transformative processes are taking place, is the individual psyche, or one might say, the field of one's consciousness.

From my own studies of Alchemical Yoga, the working with light-fire energies, I would extend this only to say that the alchemical vessel should be understood to refer *also to the physical body and energy-field*, and not merely the mental-emotional psyche. In other words, the entire set of interrelated energy-systems constituting the human being, is the vessel or *athanor* for the alchemical transformations. The human energy-systems, which can also be thought of as "personality systems," are the multi-layered vessel, container, bodies, or sheaths (*koshas* in Yoga) for the Immortal Soul, Spirit, or Essence.

Western esoteric teachings concur in asserting that there are four intermediate or personality levels of consciousness, or four bodies of differing density or vibratory frequency. The physical body (called "sheath made of food" in the Yoga tradition) is the heaviest or densest; and in order of decreasing density or increasing vibratory rate, the others are – the perceptual (or etheric), the emotional (or astral or psychic), and the mental (or noetic). Above the mental ("above" referring to vibratory rate, not space) are the three or four transpersonal levels of Soul and Spirit. Rudolf Steiner's formulation, consistent with this, is to say there are three *personal levels of soul:* the mental soul, the emotional soul and the sensory soul. In Jung's psychology, these teachings of four aspects of the human psyche are transformed into his theory of *four functions*: thinking, feeling, intuition, and sensation, which may be differently developed in individuals of different type.

Although the names may vary somewhat in various esoteric texts, on the whole there is a recognition that these four levels of the human being are related symbolically, and by resonant correpondence to the *four elements as states of matter*. The element *AIR* refers to matter in its gaseous state, to breath and breathing, and corresponds to the mental body and Jung's thinking function. The element *WATER* refers to liquids of all kinds, including fluids in the body (water, blood, lymph, hormones), and corresponds to the emotional body and the feeling function. The element *FIRE* refers to energy and radiation of all kinds, including electro-magnetic energy fields of the human nervous systems, and corresponds to the perceptual body and intuitive function. The element *EARTH* refers to material substance of all kinds, including the flesh and bones physical body, and corresponds to the sensation function, in Jung's terminology.

A moment's reflection will enable one to see that the gaseous, fluid, electro-magnetic and solid elements making up the human body, and the personality systems related to it by symbolic resonance, are always in different phases of transformation one into the other. Thoughts trigger feelings, perceptions instigate thoughts and behavior, and so on, just as solids dissolve into liquids (the alchemical *solutio*), and liquids congeal into solid matter (the alchemical *coagulatio*). Consciously participating in and amplifying these elemental transformations with intention toward a healthier, more harmonious and more integrated functioning is the alchemical spiritual healing practice, or *opus*. One traditional definition of the alchemical *opus* was that it involved *the marriage of the subtle and the dense:* the integration of the subtle psychic and spiritual energies with the dense material body. The alchemical motto *solve et coagula* ("dissolve and coagulate"), can also be understood in these terms: we should dissolve the solidified defensive structures (physical, perceptual, emotional, mental) so Spirit can be released; and solidify the energy flows of the high-frequency subtle dimensions into the material body – the process also referred to as earthing or embodiment.

In tracing the historical roots of alchemy to shamanic knowledge-seeking traditions, a question that arises is what happened to the understanding and practice of altered states of consciousness – the "shamanic journey" to acquire healing knowledge and power, which is the central technical process in shamanism. We must remember that shamanic practices arose in hunter-gatherer societies, particularly among hunters in intimate contact with animals – both those hunted for food, and those that are hunters or raptors themselves, as allies. Thus the metaphor of the journey – riding on an animal or transformed into one – is a natural choice to describe the process of seeking knowledge for healing or guidance (known as divination) by going into an intentional lucid trance state. Such shamanic journey states were typically induced by rhythmic drumming, as in Siberian and other Northern Hemisphere indigenous societies, or by the ingestion of psychoactive plant extracts, usually accompanied by rhythmic chanting, as in the ceremonies involving peyote, or the psilocybe mushroom, or ayahuasca. The use of plant extracts for shamanic journey work has been more common in tropical and sub-tropical latitudes, because of the greater diversity of plant life in those regions.

The first alchemists, by contrast, were craftsmen (they called themselves *artists*) in the fields of mining and blacksmithing, living in villages or towns. They were also health practitioners using medicinal minerals, herbs, and fungi. So their preferred term for the work of self-transformation, was in fact *opus* – "the work" or the *art*. Their interest was in long-lasting transformations of the totality of the human being. The various operations of the alchemical work are metaphors for the intentional processes of self-transformation, at the mental, emotional, perceptual and physical levels. For example, the operation called *solutio* or "dissolving," which was represented in alchemical literature by the image of a man (or a couple) sitting in a hot tub, is a metaphor for the process of dissolving the physico-psychic armoring and defensive structures that block and distort the flow of life energy. The purification of substances using fire or heat (called *purificatio*) is a metaphor for the refinement of thought and perception using the purification methods of yogic inner fire.

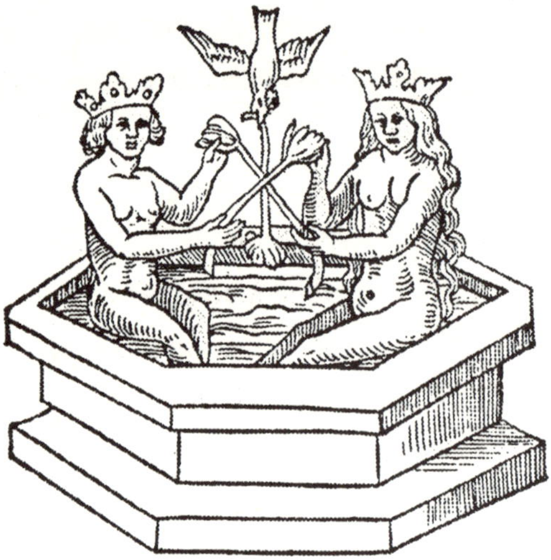

***Solutio* in the alchemical vessel.**

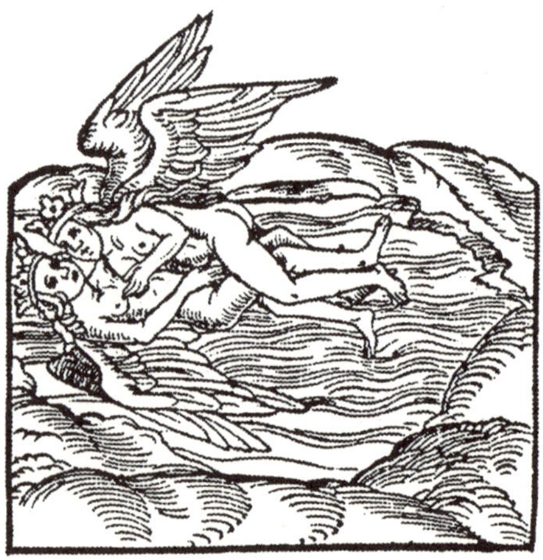

***Conuinctio* in *EARTH, WATER* and *AIR*.**

Images from the *Rosarium Philosophorum* (16th C.)

The operation of *separatio* is the analytical process of separating complex patterns into constituent elements. C. G. Jung used to say that we need to practice the "setting apart" of the contents of the unconscious (*auseinandersetzen*). The operation of *coniunctio*, the conjunction of Sun and Moon, or King and Queen, to which Jung devoted his most massive tome, is a metaphor for the integration of masculine and feminine energies, or *animus* and *anima*, within the psyche. The Jungian psychotherapist Edward Edinger, in his book *Anatomy of the Psyche,* offers insightful psychological interpretations and symbolic elaborations of these alchemical operations and others, including *calcinatio, coagulatio, mortificatio, purificatio, solutio, sublimatio, separatio*, and *conuinctio* (Edinger, 1985).

It is the great merit of Jung's work to have rehabilitated the alchemical wisdom tradition from its status as a discredited underground superstition, and to reformulate it as the symbolic language of choice for analytical depth psychology. Jung's writings aimed at establishing the reality of psychological phenomena and processes, against the exclusionary truth claims of materialist and behaviorist psychology in the first half of the 20th century. His psychology also made room for the acceptance and consideration of religious imagery, both Western and Eastern, including Yoga, Buddhism and Chinese Taoism.

It remained for another Swiss scientist of the 20th century, Albert Hofmann (a Baseler, whereas Jung was a Züricher), to reconnect psychology with the material element of the holistic alchemical tradition. With the discovery of psychoactive or psychedelic ("mind-manifesting") drugs (or perhaps we should say re-discovery, since the evidence indicates they were known in ancient times) the Western healing and spiritual knowledge tradition has come full circle from its detour through theocratic dogma and reductionistic science. The aim and practice of the Hermetic alchemical tradition is, as it ever was, the complete transformation of the individual, the physical, perceptual, emotional, mental and spiritual aspects, toward an integrated wholeness. Jung called this process *individuation* – becoming an undivided whole Self. In the symbolic language of the medieval alchemists, this process was called the quest for the philosophers' stone, the *lapis philosophorum.*

To understand the relevance of psychedelic substances to the alchemical work of holistic self-transformation, we need only remind ourselves of the research studies that have demonstrated the facilitative action of psychedelics on: (a) psychotherapy of neurotic, psychosomatic and addictive pathologies; (b) creative problem-solving and imagination; (c) growth in spiritual awareness; and (d) mystic and religious visions. The concept of psycholytic therapy, like psychoanalysis, is based on the alchemical operations of *separatio* and *solutio.* The process, whether enhanced with psychoactive substances or not, involves the setting apart of complexes into their constituent elements (thoughts, feelings, sensations, etc), and the dissolving of acquired defensive structures.

Psychedelic substances are also called "consciousness expanding" or "awareness amplifying" – the ordinarily subtle perceptions of internal states and energetic phenomena of external phenomena, like auras or energy fields, can be enormously heightened and vivified, bringing clarity and insight. Psychedelic experiences bring about an expansion of one's sense of identity beyond the usual boundaries of our body-self to an incontrovertible knowledge of one's identity as a spiritual being.

Here comes the profound relevance of psychedelic experience to a recognition of life after death, the nature of the soul, and the mysteries of incarnation. Awareness may also expand outward into a greatly enhanced sense of our interconnectedness with all life forms in the great ecological web of life, and into the greater cosmos beyond our usual Earth-centered perspective. We can come to the realization of our true identity as multi-dimensional cosmic Beings of Light.

The connection of psychedelic substances to the shamanic and yogic traditions of consciousness transformation is also evident. Albert Hofmann's own work in identifying the psychoactive principle of the visionary mushroom, and his collaboration with R. Gordon Wasson and the Mazatec shamaness Maria Sabina, made a crucial re-connection to almost forgotten shamanic traditions of the use of material biological substances in the quest for healing and knowledge. His work on the identification of the elusive secret of the Eleusinian mystery religion re-established a link to the deepest spiritual wisdom tradition of the ancient, classical world (Wasson, *et al*, 1978). The testimony of numerous practicioners of meditation and yoga has demonstrated without a doubt that the psychophysiological practices of yoga, especially tantric yoga, and the essence-path of *rasayana*, can be enormously facilitated and strengthened with the judicious and careful use of psychedelic substances (Metzner, 1998).

I want to point out here that psychedelic or entheogenic drugs by themselves do not produce healing, therapeutic or mystical experience: it is not a question of pharmacology or drug effects. Everything depends on set and setting, on intention. And awareness tools, like any tools, can be misused and abused. But given a spiritual orientation and intention they can be used to amplify, catalyze and facilitate healing, psychotherapeutic, creative and meditative processes in shamanic, yogic and alchemical practice, as well as in complementary medicine and therapy.

So what then is, or was, the Philosophers Stone and how does it relate to psychedelic, visionary, and mystical experience?[2]

First, stone is matter from the mineral realm of nature, the primordial substrate or ground of all life and therefore consciousness. We are connected with the mineral realm at the molecular level since certain of the elements in our body and in our food are mineral elements. The molecular level of reality and consciousness is more basic than the level of cellular life. One could say that if awareness is grounded at the molecular level, it is truly grounded. Perhaps this is the meaning of the expression "being stoned" that is popularly used to describe the psychedelic state. Furthermore, psychedelic drugs and endogenous neurotransmitters that induce visions and dreams in the brain, such as DMT, may take the form of purified and crystallized mineral or plant extracts.

Second, the *lapis* is also described as being fluid, like water, or an essence or tincture, or a healing panacea, or a combination of stone and water. One alchemical text of the 17th century is titled *The Sophic Hydrolith* ("The Waterstone of Wisdom"). Symbolically, this suggests that the psychedelic, visionary state of consciousness, while grounded fully in material reality, is also fluid, non-attached and flowing, like the ancient Chinese way of Tao, the watercourse way.

Third, the stone is said to be everywhere around one in external reality. "Our stone is found in all mountains, all trees, all herbs, and animals, and with all human beings. It wears many different colors, contains the four elements, and has been designated a microcosm," says the 16th century text *Glory of the World.* "This stone is under you, and near you, and above you, and around you," states another text. This is reminiscent of the saying of Jesus from the Gnostic *Gospel of Thomas:* "The Kingdom of Heaven is spread out upon the Earth, and men do not see it… The Kingdom is inside of you, and it is outside of you."

Fourth, and yet, not obvious and overt. "Our substance is openly displayed before the eyes of all, and yet it is not known," according to a text called *The New Chemical Light.* "Learned doctors…have it before their eyes every day, but they do not understand it, because they never attend to it." (*The Glory of the World*). This perhaps points to the fluid elusiveness and interiority of this water-stone consciousness – it is entirely a function of the attitude and perspective we take on things – and not something you can point out to someone else. "Those who have eyes to see will see."

Fifth, the stone is within. "This thing is extracted from you, you are its ore;…and when you have experienced this, the love and desire for it will be increased in you," according to the 17th century writer Morienus.

The experience is an inner experience, arising out of the core of our being, whether it is catalyzed by an external crystalline substance or coming to us spontaneously. It is a state of wisdom consciousness, that can only be known through direct personal experience. "We cannot be resolved of any doubt except by experiment, and there is no better way to make it than on ourselves," wrote Gerhard Dorn (18th century). My teacher of alchemical yoga Russell Schofield once told me: "The philosopher's stone is not a magical object, it is the magnificent condition resulting from reaching objectivity." The stone is the ability to be objective about fact, to perceive and know the "hard fact" of a given situation as it actually is, without illusions and distortions. To know objectively is to know with the certainty that one knows. Just as in mining, the precious stone needs to be separated from the surrounding ore that covers and conceals it, so the precious essence of truth has to be separated from the superimposed illusions and distortions.

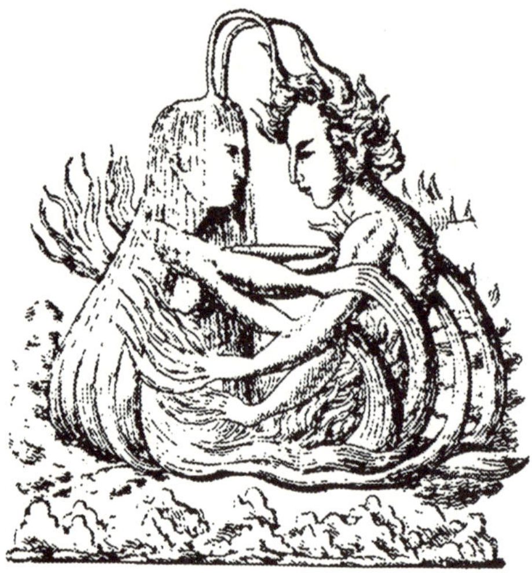

Union of *FIRE* and *WATER*

Sixth, the stone is the offspring of the inner union or *coniunctio* of Sun and Moon. "This child of the two parents, of the elements and heaven, has in itself such a nature that the potentiality and the actuality of both parents can be found in it."(Gerhard Dorn). In the legendary text *The Emerald Tablet*, attributed to Hermes Trismegistos, we read "The Sun is its Father, the Moon its Mother, the Wind bears it in its womb, and it is nursed by the Earth." *Sun and Moon* or *King and Queen* are consistent alchemical symbolic images for the basic yang-yin, dynamic-receptive, electric-magnetic polarity of the human personality and body as energy systems. Their integration in the alchemical transformation work is metaphorically portrayed as the inner marriage, or royal marriage. In Jungian terms this would be called the integration of the masculine *animus* and feminine *anima* component of the psyche. The metaphoric portrayal of this central interior process and practice as a sexual conjoining of male and female, is also found in the iconography of the Hindu and Buddhist *Tantras* and in Chinese Taoism. The Wisdom Stone is said to be the offspring or result of this inner union, i.e. the result of extended practice eliminating the obstructions to this kind of interior conjunction. The alchemical work was also often described as the *marriage of fire and water. FIRE* and *AIR* are considered masculine, because their energies rise upward and disperse outward. *WATER* and *EARTH* are considered feminine, because their energies sink downward and gather inward.

Seventh, the stone partakes of all four elements. "It is called perfect because it has in itself the nature of mineral, vegetable and animal. For the stone is triple and one, having four natures," wrote Hortulanus. "It illumines all bodies, since it is the light of the light, and their tincture," acording to Geber. "When the pure and essential elements are joined together in loving equilibrium, as they are in our Stone, they are inseparable and immortal, like the human body in Paradise" states a text called *The New Chemical Light.* This means that the state or condition

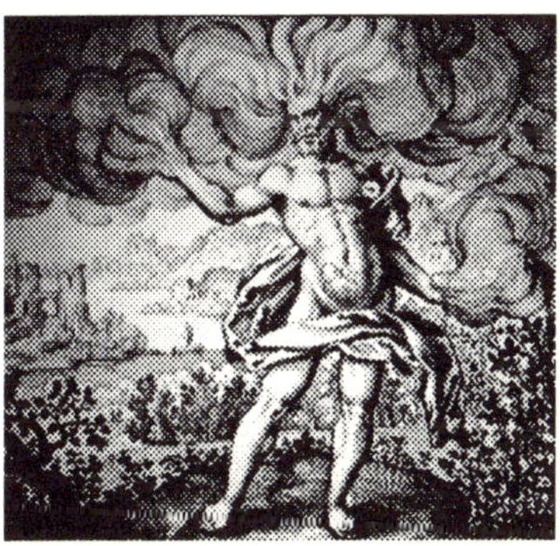

The wind has carried it in its wonb.

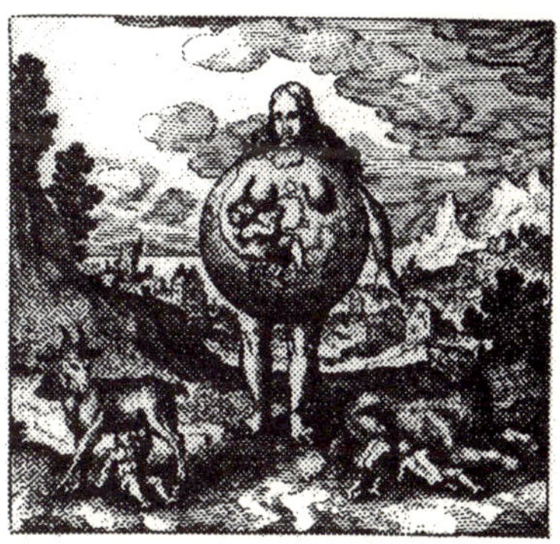

It is nursed by the Earth.

Images from *Atalanta Fugiens*, by Michael Maier, 1618

of enlightened wisdom consciousness involves the integrated functioning of all four levels of consciousness or functions – the mental-thinking, emotional-feeling, perceptual-intuitive, and physical-sensate – as well as Soul and Spirit. The alchemists would also say that this integrated functioning of all four elemental processes can produce a fifth essence *(quintessentia)*. Perhaps, this more subtle and spiritual essence corresponds to what C. G. Jung spoke of as the *transcendent function* – although I would prefer to call the fifth essence a key transformative function.[3]

From the legendary *Emerald Tablet*, a text attributed to Hermes Trismegistus, we learn that this transformative essence-stone is the offspring of the marriage of *FIRE* and *WATER* ("The Sun is its Father, the Moon is its Mother"). It is conceived and carried first in elemental *AIR*, the mind ("The wind has carried it in its womb"). It is then nourished and grounded in the physical earth-body ("It is nursed by the *EARTH*").

Finally, the Philosophers' Stone is something supremely precious and extraordinary. The text called *The Sophic Hydrolith* calls it "The most ancient, secret, natural, incomprehensible, heavenly, blessed, beatified, and triune, universal Stone of the Sages." Similar effusive praises of this rare and precious state are scattered throughout the alchemical literature of the European Middle Ages. I think it would not be an exaggeration to say that virtually everyone who has ever experienced a full-blown visionary opening produced by LSD or other psychedelics under favorable circumstances, would echo such statements. For myself, I would say that my first psychedelic experience, which was with psilocybin, in 1961, was one of the two most profound turning points in my life – after which everything in my life changed. Hardly a month goes by even now (including when I was writing this text), when I do not hear a similar sentiment expressed to me by someone, in regard to their first, and sometimes only, psychedelic experience.

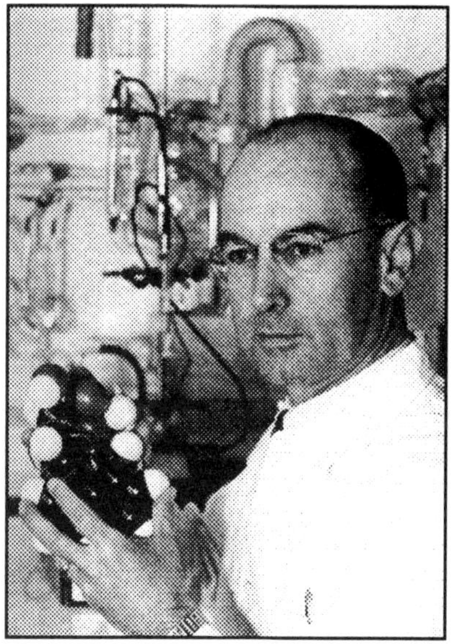

Albert Hofmann, late 1940's, with model of LSD molecule.
Photo by C. Roessiger

I would like to conclude by relating these descriptions of the miraculous properties of the Stone of the Sages, to Albert Hofmann's story of his discovery of LSD. The story is well known, and I will only mention briefly certain strange aspects, which seem to indicate some kind of divinely inspired event, a *synchronicity*, in Jung's terms. First, there is the highly significant timing of this discovery – in 1943, at the height of WWII, within months of Enrico Fermi's fist controlled nuclear chain reaction, which led directly to the building of the atomic bomb; as if it was to be a kind of psychospiritual antidote to this death weapon. Then there is the extreme improbability of a Swiss pharmaceutical laboratory chemist, having such sloppy lab techniques as to accidentally absorb a chemical through his skin! But what intrigued me the most about his story, was how Hofmann knew that the experience he was having was triggered by a drug – leading him to go back to the lab and test it out.

Although the profound consciousness-altering effects of mescaline, derived from the peyote cactus, were known, and Kurt Beringer had published studies of mescaline at the University of

Heidelberg in the 1920s, Albert Hofmann has told me he did not know this work at the time. He was a journeyman chemist and his area of expertise was the pharmaceutical chemistry of ergot alkaloids. In response to my question of how he knew it was a material substance he had ingested, he related the story from his childhood when the nine-year old experienced the oneness and all-inclusiveness of the natural world. He has described this visionary experience in his autobiographical *LSD – My Problem Child:*

> "As I was walking through the fresh green woods, suffused with morning sunlight and filled with the song of birds, all at once everything appeared in an extraordinarily clear light. Had I previously not really looked, and was I now suddenly seeing these springtime woods as they really were? They were glowing with a light that touched my heart with its beauty and seemed to draw me into its splendor. An indescribable feeling of blessed belongingness and connectedness was flowing through me." (Hofmann, 1980)

We can notice here the same language and imagery that the alchemists used when describing their experience of the stone-wisdom. As a child, he thought he would never be able to express or relate this experience through words or painting or music, and so instead decided to devote his life to the scientific understanding of the material world – to become a chemist. He realized, that day in April 1943, that the perception of the all-inclusive wholeness and belongingness with Nature he was having, must have been triggered in him by a natural material substance. That and subsequent experiences with LSD and psilocybin, led him to conclude that certain psychoactive plant substances could, under certain conditions, evoke experiences similar to this kind of spontaneous natural mystical vision. Hofmann himself has said that the deepest significance of the LSD experience goes beyond its uses as a powerful aid to psychiatry – for it points the way to a reconciliation between the scientific and the mystical worldview.

I will mention one last interesting synchronicity between Hofmann's work and the teachings of the alchemical philosophers. The alchemists said, as mentioned above, that the stone-wisdom consciousness, was the offspring of the inner conjunction of Sun and Moon, which I translate as the balanced integration of the dynamic-receptive polarity of the human energy systems. In Hofmann's philosophical writings he has formulated a theory that he calls the transmitter-receiver model of reality. I quote from his lovely little gem of a book, *Insight/Outlook*.

> "What we call reality comes into being through an interaction between outer and inner space...It (reality) is the product of a transmitter in external space and a receiver in inner space...What we call reality is the product of a reciprocal interaction between material and energetic signals being emitted from the external world and the conscious living self in the inner world of the human being." (Hofmann, 1989)

One could regard this as a philosophical statement or expression of the inner knowing of the *coniunctio,* growing out of his psychedelic experiences.

In conclusion – I am *not* saying that LSD or any other psychoactive molecule *is* the legendary Stone of the Philosophers. I am saying that through the discovery of psychedelic substances, and in particular LSD (with its extreme potency), and with his recognition of its spiritual significance, Albert Hofmann re-connected the broken thread of the West's alchemical wisdom tradition. In making his contributions to published scientific chemistry and medicine, at the time and the place in which he found himself, he provided all present and future seekers a wonderful aid in their quest for that most precious Wisdom Water-Stone, and a key to liberating self-knowledge. For that, I bow to Albert Hofmann, from the depths of my soul, with the most profound gratitude.

Notes

[1] This essay was originally presented as a talk at the conference in honor of Albert Hofmann's 100th birthday, in Basel, January, 2006; and published, in German, in Liggenstorfer, R. and Broeckers, M. (eds.) *Albert Hofmann und die Entstehung des LSD.* AT Verlag, Baden & Nachtschatten Verlag, Solothurn, 2006.

[2] The alchemical texts quoted are from the two-volume anthology *The Hermetic Museum,* restored and enlarged, transl. from the Latin, with an introduction by A.E. Waite. (London: James Elliott & Co., 1893; orig. publ. Frankfurt: 1678.)

[3] Jungians would probably not agree with my equating the transcendent function with a transformative "fifth essence." My friend and colleague Michael Flanagin comments: "The way Jung uses transcendence implies transformation, but with an added sense of creative resolution that arises from the unconscious in response to a one-sided conscious conflict…through the production of a symbol that transcends conscious limitation, creatively synthesizing the splits so that life can flow forward." (Personal communication, 2006).

References

Edinger, Edward. *Anatomy of the Psyche: Alchemical Symbolism in Psychotherapy.* La Salle, IL.: Open Court Publishing, 1985.

Eliade, Mircea. *The Forge and the Crucible.* New York: Harper & row, 1962.

Eliade, Mircea. *Yoga, Imortality and Freedom.* Princeton, NJ: Princeton University Press, 1969.

Hofmann, Albert. *LSD: My Problem Child.* Transl. Jonathan Ott. New York: McGraw-Hill, 1980.

Hofmann, Albert. *Insight/Outlook.* Transl. Dieter Hagenbach. Atlanta, GA: New Humanics, 1989.

Metzner, Ralph. *The Well of Remembrance.* Boston: Shambhala, 1994.

Metzner, Ralph. *The Unfolding Self: Varieties of Transformative Experience.* Novato, CA: Origin Press, 1998.

Sitchin, Zacharia. *The Twelfth Planet.* (First book of *The Earth Chronicles*). NY: Stein and Day, 1976.

Wasson, R. Gordon; Ruck, Carl A. P.; Hofmann, Albert. *The Road to Eleusis: Unveiling the Secret of the Mysteries.* NY: Harcourt Brace Jovanovich, 1978.

West, John Anthony. *Serpent in the Sky: The High Wisdom of Ancient Egypt.* Wheaton, Il: Quest Books Theosophical Publishing House, 1973.

Expansions of Collective Consciousness

A Brief History Since the End of World War II

The first consciousness-expanding experience, triggered by LSD, or by some other catalyst, often represents a significant transformative turning point in an individual's life. Similarly, I suggest that the introduction of psychedelics into Western culture in the mid-twentieth century catalyzed a series of profound socio-cultural transformative movements that seemed to occur synchronistically in different areas of society. These transformative expansions of consciousness may be seen as a response of the collective psyche of humanity to the unprecedented threat to civilization posed by nuclear weaponry, as well as rapidly increasing environmental devastation and runaway population growth.

In the individual, a psychedelic experience, especially the initial one, typically leads to a more or less total deconstruction of one's worldview, the model of reality and of social relations that we have come to accept through our upbringing and education. The individual may become aware of new possibilities and new choices that can be made. This expanded consciousness, or heightened self-awareness, is the basis for the therapeutic applications of psychedelics, in such areas as the treatment of addictions. Likewise, at the societal and cultural level, the consciousness expanding movements challenged the existing conventional orders, and thereby motivated groups to explore new options and energize new values. A new *culture of consciousness expansion*, initiated in the 1940s and flowering in the

1960s, lead to profound healing transformations in key areas of society over the next half century.

In WWII, human civilization had arrived at a kind of horrible climax of destructive violence, with the scope of destruction enormously amplified over previous wars by new technologies resulting from scientific advances. Over the ensuing decades, leaders and groups in all countries created new political institutions to contain the seemingly intractable tendencies to further violence; and to establish the rule of law as the basis for resolving inter-group differences. At the same time, as if in counterpoint to the nuclear death weapon and the genocidal spasm of the holocaust, the discovery of consciousness expanding drugs seemed to catalyze revolutionary changes in collective consciousness – even if and when the drugs were not directly involved in those movements.

Recent work by the philosopher Richard Tarnas, in his book *Cosmos and Psyche* (Tarnas, 2006), has shown that the cyclically changing relationships of the outer planets, when in so-called "hard" aspects (especially conjunctions, squares and oppositions), indicate deep archetypal forces being expressed synchronistically in historical and political events and cultural movements. In terms of this revisioning of the ancient science of astrology, the two planetary archetypes most closely associated with consciousness expansion are *Uranus*, when the changes involved are sudden and dramatic breakthroughs; and *Neptune,* when they are a gradual dissolving of boundaries. In addition, the planetary archetype *Jupiter* is associated with expansive values, ideals and visions; *Saturn* with contractive, stabilizing systems of order and control; and *Pluto* with explosive, propulsive forces of violent change. At the end of WWII, Saturn and Pluto were in close square aspect, symbolizing the violent destruction of the existing social order; and a Jupiter/Uranus alignment suggested momentum toward a new expansive vision. Tarnas's descriptions of the cyclical changes in society and culture complement the more linear, octave-like series of transformations that I am delineating here.

In what follows, for each decade since WWII, I intend to summarize *first* the major political and economic events, in the world and in the US, and the initiatives toward a more open and non-violent society; and *second* the new developments in culture, science and technology, that seem to encapsulate the spirit of the times and an expanding vision of the world.[1] *Third*, I will comment briefly on developments in the subculture of the psychedelic consciousness revolution, for each decade.

The 1940s

Global and US Politics

World war rages across Europe and the Pacific. Nazi Germany invades and occupies Denmark, Netherlands, Belgium, and France; and launches air war against England. Japan attacks Pearl Harbor, drawing the United States into war (1942). Once the US enters the war, the war time economy eventually lifts the country out of the Depression of the 1930s. German troops invade Soviet Russia, extending as far as Moscow. They are beaten back, as was Napoleon a century before, in part by the brutally cold Russian winter. Jews in Poland's Warsaw ghetto rise up against the Nazis, who respond by massacring thousands. Allied forces invade and defeat Italy, and Fascist Italian dictator Mussolini is killed by a mob. Allied troops storm the beaches at Normandy, under the command of General Eisenhower, and France is liberated. Roosevelt is elected to a fourth term as president of the United States (1944). Soviet troops liberate the concentration camp at Auschwitz, in Poland. An estimated 6 million Jews, as well as other minorities, disabled and dissidents, died in the German camps. In August 1945, U.S. planes drop atomic bombs on Hiroshima and Nagasaki, though Japan had already signalled it was willing to surrender, killing upward of 100,000 people instantly. World War II ends, having cost the lives of 50 million people.

The United Nations is established in 1946 at a San Francisco conference – its mission: "to eliminate forever the scourge of war." The UN General Assembly adopts a *Universal Declaration of Human Rights.* After the war, diplomatic conflict intensifies between the United States and the U.S.S.R. as an "iron curtain" is drawn across Europe and a "cold war" of influence competition and nuclear arms race commences, which dominates the world for the next fifty years. The Truman Doctrine establishes the American cold war policy of "containment" of Soviet influence. In the US, the Defense Department and the CIA are established, foreshadowing decades of increasing militarization and secret interventions by the US in destabilizing operations all over the world. Sightings of UFO's are reported with increasing frequency in the media, though always accompanied by official denial and dismissal. There is suggestive evidence (not reported till much later) that the frequency of UFO sightings is correlated with nuclear test explosions.[2]

The Marshall Plan directs massive funds to assist European economic recovery. The North Atlantic Treaty Organization (NATO) is founded, purportedly to protect Europe from imminent Soviet invasion threat. Germany is divided into two nations – becoming Soviet and American client states, respectively. India gains independence from Britain's colonial empire; millions die in riots following partition between Hindu India and Muslim Pakistan (1947). In newly independent India, Mahatma Gandhi, the apostle of non-violence, is assassinated (1948). The state of Israel is created in the Middle East, prompting decades of Arab-Israel conflict. In South Africa, racial apartheid is instituted. In China, the Civil War ends, and Communist leader Mao Zedong becomes the chairman of the People's Republic of China. In the U.S., there are race riots in Harlem and 46 other U.S. cities. But also, the Congress of Racial Equality (CORE) is founded by students, to oppose racial discrimination, using Gandhi's non-violent tactics.

Consciousness Expanding Developments in Culture, Science and Technology

Already in the 1930s, and even earlier, there had been significant expansions of the Western worldview through the work of the *cultural relativism* school of anthropologists, including Franz Boas, Ruth Benedict and Margaret Mead. They argued that we needed to abandon the ethnocentric superiority stance of Western science and scholarship toward the so-called "primitives," and instead adopt the ethnological method of "participant observation." Archaeologists too were enlarging our awareness of human origins. In 1942, Ice Age cave paintings, depicting shamanic animal themes, were discovered in Lascaux, France, and dated to 15,000 years BP (before present), vastly extending and deepening our conception of human prehistory.

The increased frequency of UFO sightings attract public and media attention, raising the possibility that Earth civilization may not be alone in the Universe. Controversial reports suggest a craft crashed in the New Mexico desert in 1947, and alien technology reverse engineered by ultra secret government programs (Corso, 1997). Reports of UFO sightings, alien contacts and secret government military cover-up programs continue over the following decades, and clearly represent, for those who take them seriously, an expansion of collective worldview.

After the war, as US veterans return home, the birth rate increases by about 20% – the "Baby Boom" generation is born. Millions of new parents read Benjamin Spock's *The Commonsense Book of Baby and Child Care*, forever changing Americans' thoughts about child care. Birth control activist Margaret Sanger founds the International Planned Parenthood Federation. In 1947, the Dead Sea Scrolls, dating from the time of Christ, are discovered near Qumran in Palestine; they belonged to the ultra-orthodox Essenes, and shed new light on the historical origins of Christianity. The invention of the transistor permits miniaturization in science and technology. Key books expressing the spirit of the 1940s were: Erich Fromm's *Escape From Freedom;* Albert Camus' existentialist classic *The Stranger;* and George Orwell's *Animal Farm*, a satirical fable about the failure of communism.

Psychedelic Subculture: Hidden Beginnings

In an astounding synchronicity, the discovery of LSD, in April 1943, occurred within months of the first controlled nuclear chain reaction by Enrico Fermi, at the University of Chicago, which lead directly to the development of the atomic bomb. Was this most profound mind-altering substance destined to provide some kind of psychological counterpart to the death weapon? When Swiss chemist Albert Hofmann discovered the consciousness expanding properties of the drug LSD, he compared the experience to his mystical experiences in Nature as a child. His discovery marks a convergence of medicinal chemistry with the ancient tradition of spiritual development known as alchemy, from which it had become disconnected in the break between science and religion in the 16th century. The first research into the possible applications of LSD was performed by the military and the CIA, as one would expect from a scientific discovery made during war time and in the immediate post-war climate of cold war confrontation. The first civilian applications were in promoting understanding of psychosis – the *psychotomimetic* model, and as an adjunct to psychoanalytic therapy, for loosening of neurotic defenses and bringing about insight – the *psycholytic* model.

In considering the significance of this birth of a modern consciousness transformation movement and its subsequent spread, we can note that Hofmann found LSD in the fungal realm. He was working on ergot alkaloids, and ergot is a fungus that infests rye and other grains. Having identified, on his own person, the profound convergence between science and religion that this substance afforded, he published his findings in the scientific literature of his profession, thereby bringing this modern version of the wisdom-stone into the light of public knowledge. Neptune and Uranus, the two planetary archetypes of consciousness expansion, were in close trine. Attended by many paradoxes and mysteries, it was as if *he had stumbled upon a remedy for an illness of civilization that we didn't know we had.*

The 1950s

Global and US Politics

The Cold War between the U.S. and the U.S.S.R heats up in Korea, with the two imperial superpowers supporting opposing sides and testing their military machinery. Joseph Stalin dies (1953) and Nikita Kruschev becomes Soviet Premier (1958). The Soviets organize the Warsaw Pact to counter the Western NATO alliance. An anti-communist uprising in Hungary is brutally put down. In the US, these are the Eisenhower years. Senator Joe McCarthy begins his paranoid anti-Communist inquisition, spreading a miasma of fear and revulsion in America. The American propaganda machine stokes up fears of nuclear bombardment. In reaction to the escalating nuclear arms race, the Committee for a Sane Nuclear Policy (SANE), an anti-nuclear protest organization, is formed, attracting support from Norman Cousins, Eugene McCarthy, Benjamin Spock and many others; it merges later with the Nuclear FREEZE movement. In Little

Rock, Arkansas, white crowds protest efforts to desegregate public schools; and in Montgomery, Alabama, a bus boycott is organized by Martin Luther King, who modeled his non-violence campaign on that of Gandhi, and galvanizes the civil rights movement. U.S. Gross National Product (GNP) triples, and favorable loans for veterans returning from the war, as well as plentiful cheap oil, lead to tremendous growth in the industrial consumer economy of suburbs and automobiles.

Prime Minister Mossadegh of Iran nationalizes the British-owned oil company BP, and is overthrown in a joint US-British operation. The coup restores the Shah to absolute despotic power, and Iranian oil to joint British-US ownership. In Egypt, revolutionaries overthrow King Farouk and establish a republic. Egypt's president Nasser nationalizes the Suez Canal, leading to the Suez crisis, an invasion of Egypt by Israel, Britain, and France. A CIA-organized coup overthrows the elected government of Jacobo Arbenz in Guatemala, precipitating 40 years of barbaric military death-squad repression and genocide against the indigenous Maya. In terms of the planetary archetypes of change, Saturnian repression and control are "squared" with Plutonic violence.

Waves of decolonization movements, dismantling the colonial governments established by European nations at the end of WWI, sweep through the African continent. Some are relatively peaceful, such as with Ghana winning independence from Britain, and Morocco from France. Others, like the Mau Mau rebellion in Kenya, drag on for years and provoke brutal reprisals, with torture and killings, from the British.

The Chinese Communists, consolidating their control over the Asian land-mass, launch an invasion of Tibet, claiming this ancient Buddhist theocracy as part of China. Thousands of lamas, male and female, are imprisoned, tortured and killed. Hundreds of monasteries and their religious arts and artifacts are destroyed. As Chinese repression intensifies to a full-scale genocide, the Dalai Lama, Tibetan spiritual and worldly leader, flees across the Himalayas to India (1959).

Consciousness Expanding Developments in Culture, Science and Technology

Alarmed by advances of the Soviet space program, the United States establishes NASA (the National Aeronautics and Space Administration). Space exploration becomes an arena of Cold War competition, hand-in-hand with military armaments competition. The first birth control pill is introduced, making management of contraception easier for millions. Francis Crick and James Watson discover the double helix of DNA, the fundamental molecular code of life. Francis Crick later states that ingestion of LSD sparked his creative insight. The polio vaccine, developed by microbiologist Jonas Salk, is declared safe for use. Just three years prior, polio had stricken over 50,000 Americans. Rock 'n Roll music becomes popular with stars like Bill Haley, Chuck Berry and Elvis Presley. Louis Leakey finds oldest hominid skull in Olduvai Gorge in Tanzania, suggesting that human evolution began on the continent of Africa, not Asia as previously believed.

Key books emblematic of the spirit of the 1950s were: Ernest Hemingway's *The Old Man in the Sea;* James Baldwin's *Go Tell It On The Mountain*; Samuel Beckett's *Waiting for Godot;* Arthur Miller's *The Crucible;* Vladimir Nabokov's *Lolita;* Allen Ginsberg's Beat classic *Howl;* Jack Kerouac's *On the Road;* Boris

Pasternak's *Dr. Zhivago;* John Kenneth Galbraith's *The Affluent Society.* Key films of the 1950s: *A Streetcar Named Desire* (with Marlon Brando); *High Noon* (with Gary Cooper). The Uranus archetype of creative breakthrough and the Neptune archetype of boundary dissolution are in close aspect.

Psychedelic Subculture: Connecting to Shamanic Roots

Applications of LSD and other psychedelics as adjuncts to psychotherapy, particularly in the treatment of alcoholism, are explored, as well as in facilitating the creative and artistic processes, in the work of Sidney Cohen and Oscar Janiger in Los Angeles. The eminent English philosopher and writer Aldous Huxley's *Doors of Perception* and *Heaven and Hell* appear in 1950; in these books he describes his experiences with mescaline as genuinely mystical, a "gratuitous grace," thus lending his enormous authority for the serious consideration of the potential spiritual significance of psychedelics.

R. Gordon Wasson rediscovers the sacred mushroom ceremony of the ancient Aztecs, publishing his account in LIFE magazine in 1957; he argues that a psychoactive plant-based visionary experience may be at the core of every religion. His account in LIFE triggers a movement in which tens of thousands North Americans and Europeans start experimenting with hallucinogenic mushrooms, at first wild and then also cultivated (Metzner, 2005). Also in the 1950s, two separate Brazilian rubber tappers start urban churches *(Santo Daime* and *Uniao de Vegetal)* in which the Amazonian shamanic entheogen ayahuasca is the central sacrament, initiating a grass-roots religious revitalization movement that now has thousands of adherents worldwide (Metzner, 2006).

Thus, in this decade, the psychedelic subculture moved beyond psychiatry into creativity and the arts, found its roots in the animistic, shamanistic traditions of indigenous cultures, and recognized its highest expression in the spiritual mystical dimensions of human existence.

The 1960s

Global and US Politics

The decade begins with John F. Kennedy being elected President of the United States, becoming the youngest and the only Catholic ever to do so. The two main geopolitical hotspots are Vietnam and Cuba. In Vietnam, the US had sided with the French after WWII, resisting Ho Chi Minh's efforts toward independence; and then became embroiled in defending the weak South Vietnam regime against what was declared to be communist take-over. In 1964, the Gulf of Tonkin incident (later revealed to have been faked) provided the pretext for a massive military build-up under President Johnson. Mounting domestic opposition to the war, as well as significant Vietcong successes, eventually led, in 1973, to American defeat and retreat from Vietnam, leaving 56,000 American soldiers and about 1.3 million Vietnamese (soldiers and civilians) dead, and the country destroyed.

In Cuba, after a revolution against the US-supported Batista regime, Fidel Castro becomes premier in 1959, and establishes political and economic ties with the Soviet Union. One of the CIA's numerous attempts to get rid of Castro ends in the Bay of Pigs invasion disaster. In 1961, when Soviet missile ships are discovered in Cuban waters, there is a tense stand-off between Kennedy and Kruschev, in which the world comes within a hairs-breadth of nuclear war. CIA resentment at perceived lack of support by Kennedy is believed by many to be one of the key motivations behind his assassination in 1963. Although never confirmed, Kennedy was also rumored to have experimented with LSD while in the White House, through his personal relationship with socialite Mary Pinchot Meyer, who befriended Tim Leary and who was herself assassinated a few months after JFK (Leary, 1983).

In the mid-sixties, the Soviets respond to democratic stirrings in Czechoslovakia by sending in tanks and troops. The Berlin Wall is built to stem the tide of refugees fleeing from East to West Berlin. In Greece, a seven-year military dictatorship begins, sponsored by the ubiquitous CIA. Algeria wins its independence from France after a bloody struggle; as Burundi, Jamaica, Samoa, Uganda and Trinidad win theirs from Britain. Other French and Belgian colonies to win their independence include Senegal, Nigeria and Congo. Leaders of former colonies who make overtures to the Soviets in their national interest, including Ghana, Nigeria and Congo, are swiftly deposed by CIA-sponsored coups and replaced by military dictators, eager to turn their country's resources over to US corporations while enriching themselves. In South Africa, African National Congress leader Nelson Mandela is sentenced to life imprisonment; his incarceration becomes a major point of contention for anti-apartheid supporters. He remains in prison for 27 years.

In China, Mao Zedong begins a Stalin-like Cultural Revolution, a purge of disaffected party leaders and intellectuals, thousands of whom are publicly humiliated, sent to labor camps or killed (1966). Japan, being forced, like Germany after the war, to build a non-military economy, becomes the world's second strongest economic power. Richard Nixon becomes president of the United States in 1969 and announces the beginning of troop withdrawal from Vietnam. He bans the use of chemical and biological weapons, and initiates Strategic Arms Limitation Talks (SALT) between the United States and the U.S.S.R., to try to get the nuclear genie back in the bottle.

Within the United States, racial tensions and violence increase dramatically during the 1960s; as do non-violent peace and racial integration movements, such as SNCC (Student Non-Violent Coordinating Committee), and the Freedom Rides in Alabama, which attempt to overturn Southern segregated voter registration and schooling. President John F. Kennedy sends federal troops to enforce integration at the University of Mississippi after rioting occurs there. In 1963, Martin Luther King, Jr., delivers his famous "I have a dream" speech, articulating a vision of an integrated society, in Washington, D.C., as more than 200,000 Americans march to demonstrate support for civil rights. The formation of the Black Panthers, a militant civil rights group evinces the increasing dissatisfaction with non-violent protest. Malcolm X, the militant spokesman for black power, is shot and killed in 1965. Civil Rights demonstrations and riots increase despite arrests, killing dozens and injuring thousands. Martin Luther King leads marches in Selma, Alabama, as well as in Chicago (1965).

In counterpoint to the escalating wars in Southeast Asia, anti-war protests and draft resistance also increase. At the University of Michigan, a "teach-in" is held to protest the Vietnam War and heralds the beginning of the student anti-war movement (1965). Martin Luther King lends his powerful voice to this struggle also, as more than 100,000 people demonstrate in New York and 150,000 outside the Pentagon. The Free Speech movement starts at UC Berkeley and sparks student protests around the country. Inspired by members of the Students for a Democratic Society (SDS) Columbia University students stage a sit-in, closing down the university in protest (1968). The Federal Bureau of Investigation (FBI) mounts an intrusively violent counter-intelligence program (COINTELPRO) against black power groups and other dissident groups. The tragic and violent climax of the decade occurs in 1968, as campaigning presidential candidate Robert F. Kennedy is assassinated in Los Angeles and Civil Rights leader Martin Luther King, Jr., is assassinated in Memphis, Tennessee (1968).

Rick Tarnas has shown that the 1960s, like other major revolutionary movements, were marked by multiple hard aspects of Uranus, Pluto and Saturn, the archetypes of liberating creativity, eruptive violence and repressive control. One of the most striking synchronicities of the decade is the following: John F. Kennedy, the charismatic President, who some believe was attempting to pull Americans out of Vietnam, is assassinated on November 22nd in Dallas, Texas (1963). Aldous Huxley, sage philosopher of the psychedelic mystical vision, *dies on the same day*, taking a 100 mcg dose of LSD for his final transition – a ceremony envisioned in his last book, the utopian novel *Island.*

Consciousness Expanding Developments in Culture, Science and Technology

In the early sixties, the first astronauts and cosmonauts are launched into space on Earth-orbiting satellites, bringing back the first dramatic photographs of the whole Earth from space. Emblematic of the aspirations for space exploration, the television series *Star Trek,* with an alien as one of the main characters, begins airing on NBC, and becomes a cult classic in American science fiction. In 1969 Neil Armstrong becomes the first man to walk on the Moon. Multiple close conjunctions and alignments of the planetary archetypes Uranus, Pluto and Saturn characterize the revolutionary, liberating and creative energies of this period.

Rachel Carson's book *Silent Spring* (1962) raises awareness of environmental despoliation and launches the American environmental movement. In 1966 the Department of the Interior publishes its first lists of rare and endangered species. Betty Friedan's *The Feminine Mystique* (1963) launches the women's liberation movement, with its "consciousness-raising" groups, arguing that women suffer from discrimination and the illusion of self-fulfillment only through their husbands. The National Organization for Women (NOW) is founded in 1966, and Congress passes a law to guarantee women equal pay for equal work. Bob Dylan produces his first album and his songs become emblematic of the civil rights and anti-war movement. British rock bands *The Beatles* and *The Rolling Stones* "invade" America and add their colorful, fresh and unique voices to the psychedelic music of the hippie culture. In 1969 the Woodstock festival draws 500,000 fans for four days of rock and roll enhanced by the ingestion of psychedelics. The gay rights movement begins in New York with the Stonewall Inn Riot

(1969). Other landmark books and films of the 1960s include Ralph Nader's *Unsafe At Any Speed*, decrying the dangers of automobiles, beginning the consumer protection movement; Theodore Roszak's *The Making of A Counterculture;* The Beatles' movie *Yellow Submarine*, and Stanley Kubrick's *2001: A Space Odyssey*, presaging the age of space exploration.

Psychedelic Subculture: Emergence and Flowering of the Counterculture

Experiences and experiments with psychedelic drugs emerge out of the psychiatric clinics and laboratories and secret groups. Timothy Leary and associates begin their research with psilocybin at Harvard University: studies are carried out and published with ordinary people in naturalistic setting, with convicts in Concord Prison Study, and with theology students in the production of mystical experiences. They publish *The Psychedelic Experience: A Manual Based on the Tibetan Book of the Dead* (Leary *et al,* 1964). In addition to Huxley, religious philosophers Alan Watts and Huston Smith testify to the authenticity of the religious/spiritual dimensions of psychedelic experience. Numerous poets, writers, visual artists and musicians explore and affirm the creativity-enhancing potentials of psychedelics. While the Harvard group focused on the psychological and spiritual implications of psychedelics, around the same period, in California, novelist Ken Kesey and his band of Merry Pranksters stage rock concert "acid tests," in which thousands of people take LSD, while listening to music and watching light-shows. Thus was born a *revolution in collective consciousness*, in which hundreds of thousands of people, perhaps millions, had one or more profound, life-changing psychedelic experiences.

Even though there is no evidence of a direct causative connection between ingestion of psychedelics and the socio-cultural transformation movements, each of them represents an expansion of collective consciousness, a transcending of existing limited conventions, attitudes and norms, similar to what is classically associated with psychedelic experiences. Thus one can justly say the sixties, the third phase in the octave progression that began in the 1940s, represent a *flowering of the counterculture and also of the culture of consciousness expansion:*

- The anti-war movement counters the American war-machine;
- The civil rights movement counters racist discrimination, in schools, housing, etc;
- The ecology movement counters environmental pollution by industrial corporations;
- The women's liberation movement counters the sexist discrimination of patriarchal attitudes and institutions;
- The sexual revolution of increased freedom of sexual expression, supported also by the contraceptive pill, counters and transcends many of the religion-bound conventions of marriage and family;
- The upsurge of creative innovation in music, the arts, fashion and literature counters and expands beyond the aesthetic forms inherited from previous generations.

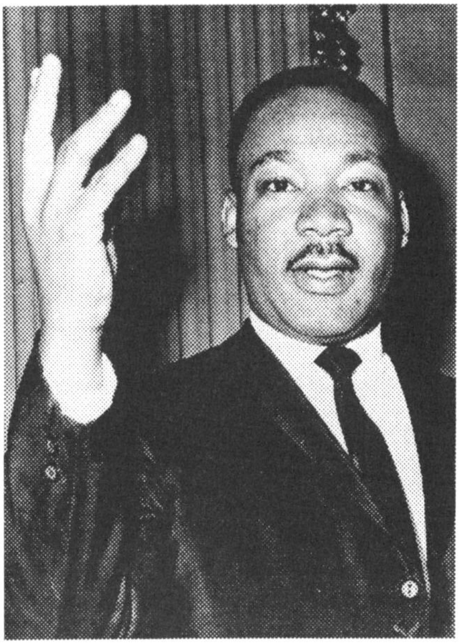

Martin Luther King (1929 - 1968)

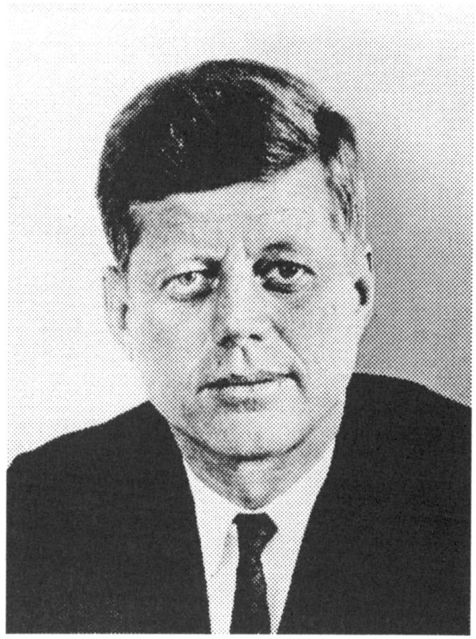

John F. Kennedy (1917 - 1963)

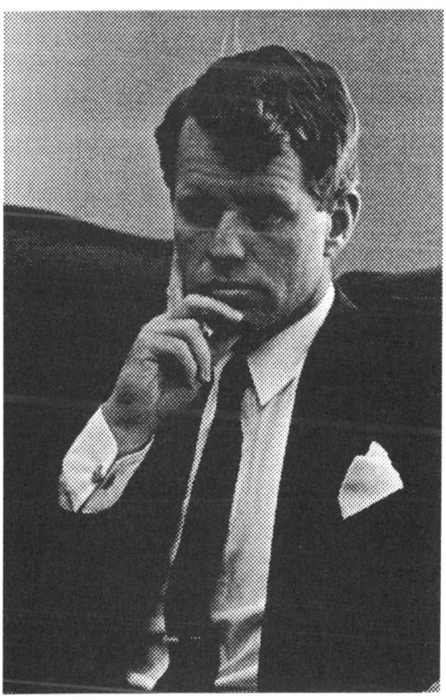

Robert F. Kennedy (1925 - 1968)

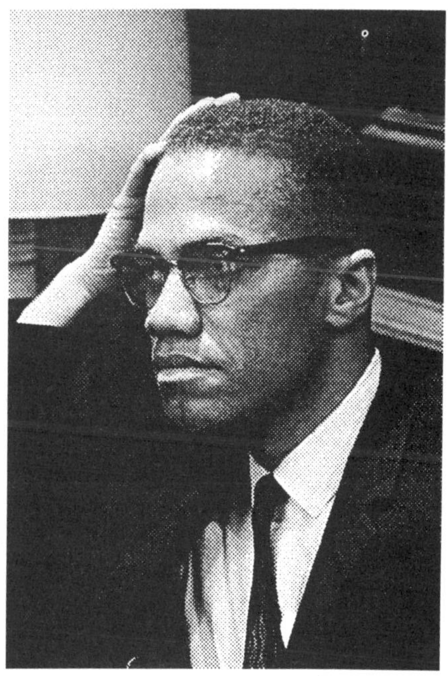

Malcolm X (1925 - 1965)

Although these social transformation movements were countercultural or even revolutionary, in that they challenged unjust, limiting or outmoded attitudes and practices of the dominant social order, it is important to *recognize that being against something was not the primary intention.* Just as, in the 19th century, waging war against the slave-holding South was not the primary intention of the abolitionist movement – rather it was the emancipation of slaves. The vision motivating the counterculture of the 1960s was pioneering innovation, reform and liberation, based on an expanded awareness of the needs of the whole society (as in the civil rights, women's liberation and sexual revolution), of all of humanity (as in the peace movement) and the entire biosphere or planet (as in the ecology movement).

As in the individual infant's struggle to be born, ultimately into a larger world and way of being, there may be a phase of intense and violent opposition to the limitations of the existing order (represented by the mother's body). This kind of opposition, which may even threaten the mother's life, is not however the ultimate aim of the neonate's struggle – which is rather to emerge from a condition that has become intolerable, too limiting, into an expanded world of greater freedom and possibilities for growth. The innovative and pioneering aspects of these socio-cultural transformations are particularly obvious in the breakthroughs that occurred from new discoveries in the sciences, and new forms of celebratory expressions in the arts. Here we don't see opposition to an existing order, but simply a highly energized, innovative and creative "moving beyond" into an expanded worldview. On the other hand, the countercultural and revolutionary elements in these movements, especially in the political and economic sphere, tends to produce violent backlash and repression by the dominant culture, as "the empire strikes back." This in turn leads to intensification of the rebellious oppositional forces, bringing about an escalation of violence and destruction – all tendencies that we can see being played out in the subsequent decades.

Undoubtedly, an energizing and amplifying influence in the growth of the consciousness culture during the 1960s was the widespread availability of inexpensive psychedelic drugs, as well as cultivated mushrooms, for personal use by increasingly large numbers of people. This certainly amplified the innovation and creativity in the arts and sciences and added much larger numbers of spiritually committed individuals to what before were relatively small minority movements. It is rumored that much of the inventiveness of the Silicon Valley high-technology companies was fueled by psychedelics including cannabis (Markoff, 2005). Drug use by musicians and artists was obvious and overt, to the point where the word "psychedelic" defined a certain genre. Whether psychedelics also amplified the rebelliousness and confrontational resistance movements is not known. Some would argue that the greater physical violence of the revolutionary movements was more connected to amphetamine use.

American society had developed into a highly stratified and diversified system, with multiple internal divisions of class, race and religion, and competing interest groups, both overt and covert. Multiple traumatic shocks to the body politic occurred during the sixties: the assassinations of two white leaders (JFK and Robert Kennedy) and two black leaders (Martin Luther King and Malcolm X). The revolutionary changes in society and culture envisioned and initiated by the counterculture, were met with violent backlash from the establishment forces of empire, domination and control. As part of this backlash, possession and use of psychedelic drugs was criminalized and all legal research on their consciousness expanding possibilities came to a halt.

Perhaps this is the impact of a very different octave series of development that also started at the end of WWII: the expansion of the global military hegemony of the American Empire. Outgoing US Republican president Dwight D. Eisenhower had warned of this development in his presidential farewell speech (1961), in which he spoke of the threat posed by the "growing and unwarranted power" and influence of the "military-industrial complex." In the light of later developments, his warning was chillingly prescient.

The 1970s

Global and US Politics

The Cold War thaws somewhat when Nixon visits the USSR and negotiates Strategic Arms Limitation Talks (SALT) I, ushering in the era of *détente.* This is formalized when 36 nations agree to the Helsinki Accords. Nixon also visits Mao Zedong in Beijing, easing decades-old American hostility towards China. In SE Asia, the American military, spearheaded by secret CIA operations, wage secret air and ground wars in Cambodia and Laos. American troops begin withdrawing from Vietnam in 1973, and by 1975, all three countries have been taken over by

Communist regimes. The Cambodian Khmer Rouge institute a reign of terror, killing hundreds of thousands of their own civilians.

In the Middle East, the Palestine Liberation Organization (PLO) stages bombing attacks against Israeli occupation forces that have expelled hundreds of thousands. Civil war rages in Lebanon betweeen Christians and Muslims. OPEC, the Middle Eastern oil-producing cartel, raises oil prices, creating energy shortages, and a recession in the latter part of the decade. Nixon delinks the US dollar from gold reserves, initiating an era of greatly increased currency speculation worldwide, as a kind of highly volatile financial bubble extends over the productive economy, a situation which has become more extreme in the decades since then. In 1974, following the Watergate scandal and its revelations of skullduggery in the White House, Nixon becomes the first US president to resign while in office. As in the 1950s, the Saturn archetype of domination and control is "squared" by the Pluto archetype of toxic violence during this decade.

In 1979, mediated by U.S. President Jimmy Carter, Egyptian President Anwar Sadat, and Israeli Prime Minister Menachem Begin sign a peace treaty – a rare event in an otherwise unrelenting cycle of violence and retribution in the Middle East. The Iranian Shah flees, and Shiite Muslim leader Ayatollah Khomeini associates take over Iran, establishing a fundamentalist Islamist state. Thousands are killed in fighting and mass executions. Also in 1979, the Soviets support a coup in Afghanistan and are drawn into a 10-year war against Mujahadeen fighters, who are recruited from Muslim countries, and enormously supported and financed by the American CIA.

Carter's security advisor Breszinski later asserted, proudly, that US support of these fighters commenced *before* the Soviet invasion, and was designed as a "trap" to lure the Soviets into their Vietnam equivalent, draining enormous human and financial resources.

In Europe, violence flares in Northern Ireland between Roman-Catholics supporting union with Ireland, and Protestants who want to remain part of the UK. Britain assumes direct control of the North Irish government. Turkish forces invade Cyprus, spurring fighting with Greek troops. The military junta resigns and Greek Premier Karamanlis returns from exile.

In Chile, in 1973, the democratically elected, popular, socialist President Salvador Allende is overthrown and killed in a CIA-backed coup. He is replaced by military dictator Pinochet, amidst widespread torture, killings and disappearances, strongly through secretly supported by the US government under Secretary of State Kissinger.

Steve Biko, an imprisoned black student leader in South Africa, dies in prison from cruelty and neglect, which leads to heightened international opposition to apartheid. South African Prime Minister Botha begins dismantling apartheid.

In the US, in 1971, two crucial events provide tipping points for popular opposition to the Vietnam War: one is the killings of four students at Kent State University in Ohio, by National Guardsmen; and the other the publication by Defense Department insider Daniel Ellsberg of *The Pentagon Papers*, a classified document detailing long-range, secretly planned U.S. involvement in Vietnam. When Carter becomes president in 1977, he pardons most draft evaders and calls them home from living abroad. Supreme Court action strengthens the civil rights movement by upholding a measure to bus children in order to enforce integration in schools. Another significant Supreme Court action, the *Roe vs Wade* decision, rules that women have the right to choose abortion. The Equal Rights amendment, guaranteeing equality for women, is passed by the Senate, but fails to be ratified by the required number of states. On Nixon's watch also, the environmental movement becomes more established in that the Environmental Protection Agency (EPA) is created by Congress to control air and water pollution; and the Endangered Species Act, which protects critical habitats, is enacted into law.

The peaking of oil production in the US in the mid-1970s, accompanied by OPEC-instigated price rises and shortages, heighten general awareness of the Western (especially US) industrial economies' dependence on Middle Eastern oil. On the one hand this provides additional agenda for military interventions around the globe, to "protect American interests." On the other hand, a positive result is that it leads to increased government support for energy conservation measures (which, in the US, is short-lived). As a symbolic demonstration, Carter installs solar panels on the White House roof, and a couple of years later Reagan has them taken down. Also on the energy front – the accident at Three Mile Island nuclear plant in 1979, which causes evacuation of over 100,000 people, heightens popular opposition to nuclear energy, and leads to a scaling back of nuclear industry expansion plans.

Consciousness Expanding Developments in Culture, Science and Technology

International cooperation in space exploration increases:

American and Soviet astronauts exchange neighborly visits when their respective satellites join in an orbital link-up. Hollywood, as so often, anticipates the future with two of the biggest blockbuster films of all time: Steven Spielberg's *Close Encounters of the Third Kind* (1977) explores the possibilities of benign encounters with alien space visitors; and George Lucas' *Star Wars* (1977) imagines wars over territory and control in the far reaches of the universe.

Expanding our knowledge of human origins backward in time, Richard Leakey and colleague find a skull in Kenya which dates the first humans to 2.5 million B.C.

Alex Haley publishes his novel *Roots* (1976), which deepens collective awareness of the slave ancestry narrative of African-Americans. Word processors and fax machines begin to populate offices. Apple Computer company launches the first personal computers – an Age of Digital Connectivity begins.

During the 1970s, several of the countercultural and consciousness expanding transformation movements that were initiated in previous decades (anti-war, civil rights, feminist, environmental, liberalization of sexual attitudes) achieved some limited success in entering the public policy realm and mainstream culture. However, the forces of repressive state power and the military-industrial complex also became stronger and more pervasive, particularly in the are of drugs and drug policy. The Nixon gang launches the "war on drugs" – possibly because the demise of McCarthy's "war on communism" left them without an internal enemy, which is a core requirement for a fascist-leaning state. Reagan and every U.S. president since then (with the possible exception of Carter) has continued and escalated these prohibitionist policies, playing up people's fear and ignorance and doing nothing to actually stop the flow of drugs into the country, nor anything to treat addiction. The criminalization of all non-medical drug use stokes a vast underground economy of interconnected narcotics trafficking gangs, drug law enforcement agencies and paramilitary gangs in other countries, especially in Latin America. The profits laundered from these operations – estimated by some to be in the hundreds of billions of dollars every year – flows back into the banking system and government coffers in the "black budget" category (Scott, 2003).

Transpersonal and spiritual perspectives begin to enter into the writings of pioneering scientists and philosophers, formulating new paradigms that expand the boundaries of the Newtonian-Cartesian worldview of Western science. I am thinking here of the work of such as Fritjof Capra, Stanislav Grof, Arthur Young, David Bohm, Buckminster Fuller, Ilya Prigogine, Rupert Sheldrake, James Lovelock, and others (Grof, 2000). New, more radical philosophical perspectives on environmentalism, such as deep ecology, social ecology, ecofeminism, bioregionalism and ecopsychology, are discussed, debated and published (Metzner, 1999).

Psychedelic Subculture: Deepening and Spreading

The scheduling of psychedelic drugs as controlled substances with no recognized medicinal value, brings all official research with these substances to a halt. Possession and use of these drugs is criminalized, on a par with heroin, cocaine and marijuana. Prohibitionist policies now cover the new psychedelic drugs as well, although the number of users is less than 10% of cannabis users, and less than 1% of users of narcotics. Because of increased government repression, many individuals in the psychedelic movement pull back from involvement in overt politics, as well as from government-approved research on the therapeutic applications of psychedelics. The effect of the multiple shocks of assassinations of charismatic leaders in the 1960s, as well as prison sentences on movement leaders including Timothy Leary, and the violence and criminality associated with LSD by the Manson gang and the Hells Angels, is to induce profound soul-searching. The intentional use of drugs and visionary plants for healing, for therapy and for spiritual growth goes underground, retreats into the private sphere. Musicians, artists and writers, inspired by their visionary experiences, continue to practice their craft and publish their work.

Other teachings and methods of consciousness-development, such as Asian yoga, Zen Buddhism and other meditation systems, many new forms of transpersonally-oriented experiential psychotherapy, New Age spiritual practices, neo-shamanic and neo-pagan interests are cultivated and become academically more respectable, through the writings of scholars and translators and immigrations of Asian teachers. The "Buddhist Dharma comes to the land of the Red Man," as the ancient Tibetan prophecy foretold. The anthropologist Michael Harner describes, in his book *The Way of the Shaman* (Harner, 1980), core techniques and perspectives of shamans worldwide – and starts to teach people the principles of shamanic journeying with a rhythmic drum beat.

The 1980s

Global and US Politics

The 1980s are the years when the Communist Soviet empire and its grip on Eastern European client states comes non-violently apart. In the early years of the decade, the Polish Solidarity Party, led by Lech Walesa, becomes the first independent labor union in the sphere of Soviet Communism. Under the leadership of Mikhail Gorbachev as general secretary of the Communist Party in the USSR, economic reforms and policies such as *glasnost* (openness), and *perestroika* (restructuring), open up the Soviet Union. In 1985, Gorbachev and Reagan sign the INF Treaty in Washington, D.C., agreeing to reduce their nuclear stockpiles. Then cascading waves of secession make former client states, including Poland, East Germany, Czechoslovakia, Hungary, Lithuania, Ukraine, Bulgaria and lastly Romania non-violently independent. The dismantling of the Berlin wall, painful emblem of Cold War enmity, in 1989, is accompanied by a jubilant free flow of humanity across a 40-year old divide. The Russian economy goes into a tailspin, social welfare systems collapse, and the infrastructure of an industrialized society crumbles. In the world's worst nuclear accident, the Chernobyl plant in the Ukraine explodes (1986), making the surrounding area a radioactive wasteland for the indefinite future, causing thousands of deaths and more thousands of disfiguring radiation sickness and birth defects.

In the US, the 1980s are the years in which Hollywood actor and Republican Ronald Reagan, elected President in 1980 and re-elected in 1984, launches a supply-side economic program which enables the U.S. economy to emerge from the recession of the late 1970s, but at the expense of explosive growth of the national deficit. Under Reagan in the US, and Margaret Thatcher in Britain, the capitalist so-called "free market" policies of privatizing and commodifying essential social services are increasingly spread throughout the Western world. Tens of millions of U.S. citizens lose their savings as numerous large savings and loan institutions fail. Independent investigators have concluded that the savings banks failures were engineered to effect a massive transfer of wealth from the working class to the wealthy elites. The War on Drugs, concentrated on heroin and cocaine, is greatly expanded under Reagan, leading to explosive growth of prison populations. The association of these drugs and narcotics trafficking with the Vietnam war and Latin American wars respectively, is reported by some courageous journalists, but not by the mainstream media (Scott, 2003). The use of "drug-war" rhetoric to amplify a climate of fear in the general population (not the actual drug users of course, but everyone else), serves to propagandize the increasing repressive social control mechanisms and widespread loss of trust in the social contract.

Under Reagan, Christian fundamentalists gather tremendous power and influence in the Republican party and increasingly dominate the media and terms of public discourse. James Watt, Reagan's Secretary of the Interior, is an avowed believer in Armageddon scenarios as are millions of others, believing environmental catastrophe are welcome signs of the impending triumphant return of the "Lord." Consequently the progressive energy conservation and environment preservation policies of the Nixon and Carter years are scaled back. Symbolically, Reagan removes the solar panels on the White

House roof installed under Carter, channeling massive subsidies to the oil and auto industry instead. These policy directions are set to continue, more or less openly through the next two decades, and are openly ascendant under the G. W. Bush regime in the White House. Synchronistically, in a darkening way, in 1989 ten million gallons of oil pollute Alaskan waters and wildlife when the *Exxon Valdez* runs aground – it is the world's worst oil industry disaster that will take years to clean up.

In the Middle East, violence re-ignites between the PLO and Israel in an Arab-Israeli war. War rages for between Iran and Iraq, with the US funding and supporting Iraq overtly and Iran covertly. A bombshell lands in American politics when it is discovered that the U.S. is selling arms to Iran during its war with Iraq and using the profits to fund Contra forces in Nicaragua. Congress investigates the Iran-Contra affair. Parts of the "black budget" operations of the CIA see the light of day, but the information is swiftly and efficiently concealed and neutralized. The Iran-Iraq war ends in 1988, after 8 years and 1.5 million dead.

After the Sandinistas come to power in Nicaragua and make peace overtures to the U.S., American policy continues to support the Contras in their revolt against the Nicaraguan government (1985). Allegations, with evidence, surface that Central American military operations, including the Contra war and death squad operations in several countries (Guatemala, Honduras, Nicaragua, Columbia) are supported by U.S.-CIA weapons and training, and funded in part by "black budget" narcotics traffic. The pattern in these countries is the same: the slightest movement toward popular democracy or even national interest, with a lessening of colonial ties to US corporations, is met with official resistance, and eventually violent repression of popular and indigenous resistance. In the end, the wealthy land-owning elites still remain in power, supported by the US, and the poor remain poor and helpless.

At the end of the decade, in 1989, Chilean voters elect Patricio Aylwin president, ending the brutal military regime of General Pinochet. Inter-religious violence erupts in India and triggers state violence when Prime Minister Indira Gandhi sends troops to the Sikh Golden Temple in India, over 500 civilians are killed. In China unprecedented huge and persistent student protests lead to a non-violent occupation of Tiananmen Square – which is brutally put down by authorities with over 1,000 unarmed protesters killed.

Summarizing, in the 1980s, the Soviet empire and its version of bureaucratic communism begins to unravel; whereas the American financial-industrial empire consolidates its economic grip on the domestic population, and militarily on overseas client states.

Consciousness Expanding Developments in Culture, Science and Technology

In 1981, *Voyager I*, a NASA probe, explores Saturn. The first space shuttle *Columbia* is launched and completes its first mission in space. But, in a major set-back for the US space program in 1986, the space shuttle *Challenger* explodes after lift-off, killing the eight astronauts aboard.

AIDS begins to be recognized as an epidemic and the rise of AIDS puts a corrective brake on the sometimes reckless exuberance of the sexual revolution. The gay sub-culture is motivated to develop vigorous new forms of social activism as well as deeper awareness of sickness, death and healing. In addition to AIDS, the 1980s and subsequent decades see the increasing spread of new infectious diseases, including Ebola, Lyme disease and SARS. Because of ever greater numbers of people living in desperately impoverished conditions, and the increasing amount of global travel, it's increasingly easy for disease vectors to spread.

Many of those identified with the counterculture of the 1960s and 1970s move to the underground, in both the private and community sphere. The movements continue to deepen, diversify and develop, reaching into all sectors of society, including the academic world, education and religions. There are radical environmental/ecological movements, such as deep ecology, ecofeminism, bioregionalism, ecopsychology, that challenge the anthropocentrism of conventional worldview. A spectrum of feminist, civil rights and social justice movement develops and become increasingly active in politics. Transpersonal psychology develops a language of spiritual experience and values free of the concepts of particular religious systems. Asian spiritual teachings, such as Indian Yoga, Zen, Tibetan Buddhism and others flourish and many Asian teachers settle and teach in the West. Such movements are recognized as contributing to a lessening of social ills and a heightening of social conscience, concern and activism. Astrologically, during the 1980s, the beneficent expansiveness of Jupiter is aligned with the liberating creativity of Uranus.

Landmark books and films that symbolize the spirit of the 1980s, are: Steven Spielberg's *E.T.* – a unique and powerful story built upon the premise of a visit by a non-threatening advanced alien species; John Huston's *The Dead* - based on a James Joyce story, the last testament of the Irish master filmmaker; and two books by African-American women – Alice Walker's *The Color Purple* (1982) and Tony Morrison's *Beloved* (1987) – both powerful narratives of the black woman slave's story under dual racist and sexist oppression; Salman Rushdie *The Satanic Verses* (1988) – a satirical novel on Islam, that garnered an Islamist death warrant for its author.

Psychedelics Subculture: Empathogens and Entheogens

For mainstream culture, the use of psychedelics has become a minor footnote in the so-called War on Drugs. Use of the classical psychedelics for purposes of healing and psycho-spiritual grown remains almost invisibly underground. Marijuana is, and remains, in the middle and hotly contested ground: life-saving and mind-assisting medicine for millions, taboo issue for the political class.

Chemist Alexander Shulgin creates the phenethylamine compound MDMA, which is found to be a uniquely valuable adjunct to psychotherapy. Unlike other psychedelics, it expands the emotional band of awareness only, leaving physical perceptions unchanged, and generating a state of empathy (hence "empathogens"), akin to meditative equanimity and emotional balance. Due to its euphoriant quality, the drug spreads from the therapists' couch to the street, becomes demonized and illegal, thereby repeating the pattern of LSD in the 1960s: initial reports of positive results in psychotherapy result in its popularization and then criminalization – on exaggerated and dubious evidence (Holland, 2001). Rave dance parties of thousands, involving

MDMA (now known as "Ecstasy"), as well as techno music and light-shows, begin in England, spread to the US, Europe and around the world. These new Dionysian revels spread throughout the suburban middle-classes as well as youth culture, recreating something of the celebratory, sensual and life-affirming ethos of the 1960s. Alignments between the liberating energy of Uranus and the mystical, boundary-dissolving archetype of Neptune, characterize this era.

The visionary mushroom culture, particularly associated with the 1960s California rock dance-band *The Grateful Dead*, as well as the ayahuasca religions, like the *Santo Daime* and *Uniao de Vegetal*, that originated in Brazil in the 1950s, continue to gather followers and spread internationally. The term *entheogens* ("connecting to the sacred within"), comes into use to describe shamanic sacraments from indigenous cultures, like peyote, psilocybe mushrooms and ayahuasca. At the end of the 19th century, the use of the peyote had become integrated into the Native American culture as a religious sacrament; now, at the and the end of the 20th, ayahuasca churches, originally from Brazil, appear to be following that same path in the US and Europe.

In the *Santo Daime* church, the entheogenic sacrament is ingested in group ceremonies involving singing and dancing; the empathogenic Ecstasy is taken in large groups at Rave dance parties; and a primary setting for the visionary mushroom continues to be the Grateful Dead dance concerts. As in the Dionysian religion of the ancient world, ecstatic consciousness expansion is associated with music and dance. The large-scale use of substances which are unacceptable and prohibited in mainstream society, has moved underground, spreading invisibly like fungal mycelium, generating non-hierarchical, informal, international networks of participatory, Earth-honoring, and life-affirming celebrations.

The 1990s

Global and US Politics

The Soviet Union officially ends, as Baltic and Central Asian republics declare their independence, the Communist party is stripped of its power, and Boris Yeltsin (and later, Vladimir Putin) becomes president of the newly reconstituted Russia. Secessionist guerilla wars in Chechnya continue, probably fueled by Western interests in an oil pipeline. Under the influence of Western capitalist "free market" racketeers, the ruble is devalued, the industrial economy implodes, the incomes of most ordinary Russians drop precipitously, and large parts of the economy devolve into black market and barter exchanges.

The collapse of the Soviet empire leaves the U.S. as the "sole superpower," increasingly nakedly dedicated to economic and military hegemony around the globe. As part of that imperialist project, President Bush the Elder, sends 400,000 troops to Saudi Arabia in 1991, using an Iraqui annexation of Kuwaiti oil fields as the pretext for establishing a power base in the region. In addition, the US/UN power group imposes crippling sanctions on Iraq, which over the next decade cause thousands of deaths of civilians and severely weaken the economy and infrastructure.

Attacks on American embassies orchestrated by Islamist terrorist groups under the command of Osama bin Laden, originally a CIA asset recruited to help drive the Soviets out of Afghanistan, lead to retaliatory air strikes against Afghanistan and Sudan. In a major setback to the Israel-Palestine peace process, Israeli Prime Minister Yitzhak Rabin is assassinated by a right-wing student angry at Rabin for turning over some land to Palestinian control.

In the US, the 1990s are the Clinton years, as the former Governor of Arkansas is elected in 1992 and again in 1996. Bill Clinton survives an attempt by the Republican controlled congress to impeach him for lying about a White House sexual affair. Issues of sex and race play a big part in US politics in this decade. The U.S. Senate approves the nomination of Clarence Thomas, an African American to the Supreme Court despite allegations by Anita Hill, also an African American law professor, of sexual harassment.

Race riots erupt in Los Angeles after white policemen are acquitted by an all-white jury of beating Rodney King, a black man, in a videotaped incident. And black football hero O.J. Simpson is acquitted of the murders of his wife Nicole and her friend Ronald Goldman, in a racially tinged sensationalist murder trial. The verdict triggers nation-wide debates about race, wealth, and the American criminal justice system.

The decade is also marked by spectacular acts of violence and destruction in the US: Federal agents raid and lay siege to the ranch of the Branch Davidian cult in Waco, Texas; the siege ends when federal agents storm the compound, which becomes engulfed in flames, killing dozens inside. The bombing of the Murrah Federal building in Oklahoma City, apparently by members of right-wing white supremacist militias, kills 168 people. Two teenage students on a vengeful murder spree kill 15 and wound 23 in Columbine High School in Littleton, Colorado in 1999.

On the non-violent side of the ledger, the collapse of Soviet rule over East Germany leads to re-unification of the two Germanies for the first time since World War II. Further Cold War thawing occurs with a Conference of Security and Cooperation in Europe, and the reduction of NATO and Warsaw Pact forces. A fragile flowering of peace occurs in Northern Ireland, when the Good Friday Accord is signed after 22 months of negotiations and 30 years of violence.

The Federal Republic of Yugoslavia, created in 1918, disintegrates, at first peacefully, as Slovenia and Croatia declare their independence and are soon followed by Bosnia, Hercegovina, and Macedonia. However, Serbian President Milosevic, hanging on to power, resists the devolution of Kosovo and Albania, and the intervention of Serbian militias escalates into civil war, marked by ethnic cleansing campaigns against Muslim populations. Supported by US aerial bombing campaigns, NATO goes to war against what remains of Yugoslavia in a three and a half years war, which claims 20,000 lives.

In Haiti, the long-standing dictatorships of Duvalier father and son end, when former priest Jean-Bertrand Aristide becomes Haiti's first democratically elected populist president. El Salvador's decades-long civil war ends when government and rebel leaders sign a pact. Signed by Canada, Mexico, and the U.S., the North American Free Trade Agreement (NAFTA) establishes the world's largest trading bloc. On the day after signing, the Zapatistas rebellion begins in Chiapas, Mexico, protesting the continued exploitation of indigenous lands and local communities, for the profits of multinational corporations. The Mexican economy teeters on the edge of bankruptcy as the peso collapses, leading to a $20 billion dollar bail-out by the US.

In South Africa, Nelson Mandela is released from prison after serving 27 years, laws of apartheid are repealed and the first multiracial free elections are held, leading to the triumph of the African National Congress and the election of Nelson Mandela to the presidency. The relatively non-violent demise of the apartheid regime is credited to a large extent to the international grassroots disinvestment campaign – pressuring individuals and institutions to withdraw investment funds from South African subsidiaries. The U.S. government had been a steadfast supporter of the apartheid regime.

In Central Africa, the presidents of Rwanda and Burundi die in a plane crash near Rwanda's capital, and this provides the pretext for a civil war between Hutu and Tutsi tribal groups. A state-supported genocide ensues as over 800,000 Tutsis are massacred in the space of a couple of months by the majority Hutus. Refugees flee the violence into neighboring Zaire, Burundi and Tanzania.

In East Timor, during a UN-sponsored referendum, the people vote to be independent of Indonesia, sparking retaliation by the Indonesian military (armed and trained by the US), who invade the tiny island nation and massacre 200,000 people, or one-third of the population. In India, thousands of Hindu extremists destroy a mosque, igniting two months of Hindu-Muslim rioting that claims thousands of lives.

On the planetary scale, *El Niño*, a large-scale periodic warming of the tropical Pacific Ocean, affects the world climate, upsetting normal weather patterns. Hurricane Mitch pounds the Caribbean and Central America, killing thousands and wiping out much of the infrastructure that had taken years to build.

Summarizing the 1990s decade, we saw multiple explosions of nationalistic and ethnic violence, as well as astonishing examples of peaceful devolution of imperialist systems – in the Soviet Union, and in South Africa. The giant multinational corporations push for more and more unhindered movement of capital and access to markets, misnamed "free trade." The Western corporate domination project, especially of the petroleum economy, are backed up by military intervention. Increasing numbers of voices are heard critical of economic globalization and the gross inequalities and exploitation of human and natural resources associated with it. The "Battle of Seattle," in 1999, is the first of a series of major street protests against the ever-increasing economic domination and exploitation by multi-national corporations and their allied governments. Scientists' warnings of multiple mounting global environmental disasters (climate change, species extinction, overpopulation, pollution, deforestation, exhaustion of resources) spread increasingly into the collective consciousness.

Consciousness Expanding Developments in Culture, Science and Technology

Several historic advances in space exploration take place during this decade: The shuttle *Discovery* is launched from Cape Canaveral, carrying the Hubble Telescope, which starts to send back dramatic never before seen photographs of cosmic objects and events. The first rendezvous of a NASA spacecraft with the Russian space station *Mir* occurs; and the NASA probe *Pathfinder* lands on Mars.

The Internet Society is chartered, and 1,000,000 host computers are connected in a network, beginning unprecedented explosive global growth of interconnectivity over the next decades. The dizzying rise and spread of the internet fosters global communications in every area of life, from crime and commerce to science, education, information (including information about drugs) and activist solidarity. Informed sources aver that many of the most creative innovators in the internet and digital technology revolution were inspired by their psychedelic drug experiences in the 1960s (Markoff, 2005).

Films epitomizing the spirit of the 1990s are: Kevin Costner's *Dances With Wolves*, which honors the legacy of the Native Americans and the tragedy of the loss of their culture in the 19th century; and Steven Spielberg's *Schindler's List*, which honors victims of the Nazi-Jewish holocaust and the courage of one individual to resist genocidal leadership.

Psychedelic Subculture: Integrating into the Internet

Prohibitionist drug war policies continue, defying logic, justice and common sense, leading to the imprisonment of hundreds of thousands, disproportionately black, individuals, for the victimless crime of possession of marijuana. Prohibition and the propaganda campaigns associated with it do nothing to stop the importation or use of drugs, or solve the public health problems associated with drug abuse. The United States is increasingly isolated in comparison to other Western nations, where the focus is more and more on *harm reduction* and common sense in relation to drug use. The drug war creates a climate of fear in the general population and increases the power of the prison-industrial complex. Prohibition and the fear associated with it fosters contraction of consciousness, and psychedelics become publicly taboo. Work with consciousness expanding methods (drug or non-drug) continues only in the underground, private sphere.

The psychedelic underground continues, becomes more knowledgeable, with clearer intentionality toward healing, therapeutic and spiritual values. Shamanic practices, work with animal, plant and spirit allies, herbal and natural medicine, organic farming and nutrition – all expand vigorously. New, more conscious, non-medical, family and home-based approaches to birth and birthing, and death and dying, gain more adherents. Alternative medical systems gain in acceptance, especially homeopathy, Chinese acupuncture, Indian ayurveda and indigenous herbal healing systems. A living systems worldview, that emphasizes interconnectivity and mutual causality, rather than atomistic, linear determinism, emerges in philosophical scientific circles, especially in the work of such thinkers as Ervin Laszlo, Fritjof Capra and Joanna Macy. The worldview of interconnectivity resonates with ancient animistic indigenous teachings in which the cosmos, and all its components, are seen as living, conscious beings.

The New Century (2000-2005)

Global and US Politics

In the 2000 American election, Republican George W. Bush, running against Al Gore, loses the popular vote but wins the majority votes of the electoral college. A disputed recount process in Florida is aborted by the U.S. Supreme Court, effectively handing the election to Bush. Many Americans see this as a court-sponsored *coup-d'état*, bringing into power the extreme right wing of the Republican party, allied with fanatical Christian fundamentalists. Advocates of a neo-conservative, imperial role for the US in world affairs, assume top positions in the new government and begin to promulgate their agenda: abrogating international treaties on nuclear arms control, undermining international and domestic laws on environmental protection, reducing the effectiveness of the United Nations, increasing military spending and claiming the right to wage pre-emptive war anywhere, any time.

On September 11, 2001, in the worst attack on American soil since Pearl Harbor, hijacked airliners slam into the twin towers of the World Trade Center in New York City, creating an explosion and fire, followed by the collapse of both towers, and a nearby third tower, in what was believed to be a coordinated terrorist attack on the United States. More than three thousand people die. Shock and fear grip the nation. The government declares that the attacks were carried out by a Muslim Arab terrorist network known as Al Qaeda, under the leadership of Osama bin Laden. The president unilaterally declares "war on terrorists," and divides the world into those "for us" and those "against us," identified as "axis of evil." Under the guise of protecting "homeland security," a systematic dismantling of constitutional rights and protections begins, accompanied by a barrage of fear-mongering propaganda, and the quashing of dissent by threat and ridicule. The 9/11 attacks were used to justify the waging of war against Afghanistan and Iraq, just as the bombing of Pearl Harbor was used to justify America's entry into World War II, and the burning of the Reichstag in 1932 was used by Hitler to launch his police state regime.

Questions were raised, that have never (as yet) been resolved, about official prior knowledge or complicity in the attacks. Research questioning the official explanation of the Trade Towers attack continues to accumulate, forcing the government to appoint an official 9/11 commission which releases its report in 2004. Dissenting voices point to numerous inconsistencies and critical ommissions in the report, leading serious researchers to conclude that the whole attack was in fact an inside job, masterminded by shadow power groups within the US establishment, possibly allied with intelligence agencies of some other countries, like Israel and Pakistan (Ruppert, 2004; Griffin and Scott, 2007). Like the continuing unresolved questions about the Kennedy assassination, this issue remains a festering open wound in the collective psyche of the American people.

In the 2004 election, Bush wins against Senator John Kerry, in a very close vote dogged by persistent charges of fraudulence in the voting process and machinery. These questions have also been extensively debated and researched, and to this day, not satisfactorily resolved – leading a sizeable number of the population to believe that the electoral process may have become irreparably corrupt and fraudulent.

For Christian fundamentalists, America's invasion of Iraq and the consequent brutal slaughter of thousands of innocent civilians in that country, are all part of a grand divine plan that will culminate in Armageddon and the establishment of an American Christian empire that will extend all over the globe. Christian fundamentalists are today among the most fanatical supporters of the neoconservative global imperialist agenda.

In Russia, President Vladimir Putin, former head of the KGB, is elected president. He consolidates central power, shifting the Russian government toward more autocratic rule. The bloody Russian struggle with Chechen Muslim separatists continues. The United States, having engineered the expulsion of the Russians from Afghanistan with the help of CIA-funded *mujahadeen* (when Osama Bin Laden was a CIA asset), begins a devastating bombing campaign on that country, ousting the fundamentalist Taliban regime, and securing an oil pipeline from Central Asian countries to the sea. The pretext for the US-led attack was that Osama bin Laden and his Al-Quaeda gang, the supposed mastermind of the September 11 terrorist attacks, were said to be hiding in Afghanistan. It was soon revealed that Afghanistan was just the first step in a campaign to extend American hegemony over areas with strategic resources, especially oil. A much bigger prize – Iraq – was soon to fall prey to America's global domination ambitions.

The rationale for the 2003 U.S. invasion of Iraq – that Iraq possessed weapons of mass destruction, and that they supported the Al Qaeda network – had, by 2005, been thoroughly discredited. The real agenda behind the invasions of Afghanistan and Iraq is widely seen, throughout the world, as being the securing of oil fields (in Iraq) and distribution pipelines (in Afghanistan), for American and Western corporate interests. Additional American interest in the invasion of Afghanistan was to re-establish the flow of opium production, which had been suppressed by the Taliban, and which has reached new peaks since their ouster. Research by Peter Dale Scott and others has documented the significant role of the international drug trade in financing secret CIA paramilitary operations in Afghanistan, as well as in Latin America and previously in Vietnam (Scott, 2003). Independent researchers and rare whistleblowers become the voices of conscience in a situation where national governments are increasingly intertwined with and manipulated by multinational corporations and their allied shadow power groups operating totally outside the established frameworks of law and political institutions.

In the Middle East, blood continues to be shed. The Israeli occupation of former Palestinian lands continues, condemned and censured by most countries and the UN, but supported and funded by successive US government, and allied Christian fundamentalist groups. Palestinian popular resistance to the occupation and counter-attacks by suicide bombers also continue. More genocidal campaigns erupt in in Africa: Janjaweed, a government-backed Arab militia in Sudan, are accused of an ethnic cleansing campaign against black Africans in Darfur. An estimated 70,000 civilians have been killed and approximately 1 million left homeless.

A deadly new respiratory virus called SARS, starting in Southern China in 2003, and the spread of avian flu, also in China in 2005, stokes fear of global flu pandemics. Public health researchers have warned for years that the accelerating pace of global interconnectedness, and the development of bacteria and viruses resistant to antibiotics, is likely to lead to hosts of new plagues. The AIDS plague continues to spread, with Africa the place with the largest number and fastest growing number of HIV-infected people, including tens of thousands of AIDS orphans.

Africa is also the continent with the most widespread and devastating levels of poverty and famine. The UN food agency issued a warning to the world that more than 38 million people in Africa are facing the prospect of famine. A report issued by the agency claimed that as of December 2002, 18 million people were at risk of starving in Ethiopia, Eritrea and Sudan.

In 2002, California experienced serious energy shortages and blackouts, precipitating an energy crisis. Later, this crisis was found to have been the result of profiteering in the deregulated "free" energy market by corporate energy giant Enron – whose principals were convicted of fraud, as thousands of employees lost their retirement savings. In 2003, blackouts hit major cities in the Eastern U.S. and Canada, leaving millions without power for periods of time ranging from a few hours to over a day. Periodic outbreaks of energy shortage, as well as rising gasoline prices, begin to raise more serious public awareness of the unprecedented phenomenon known as *Peak Oil – the unavoidable and irreversible decline of world petroleum production.* Since petroleum is the basic life-blood of industrial civilization, this peak of production, variously estimated to occur within the next 10 to 30 years (though some experts say even sooner), has catastrophic implications. In February 2005, a special report, known as the Hirsch report, commissioned by the US Dept of Energy, asserted:

> The peaking of world oil production presents the US and the world with an unprecedented risk management problem. As peaking

> is approached, liquid fuel prices and price volatility will increase dramatically, and without timely mitigation, the economic, social and political costs will be unprecedented. Viable mitigation options exist on both the supply and demand sides, but to have substantial impact, they must be initiated more than a decade in advance of peaking (Heinberg, 2004).

The global energy crisis is unfolding against a backdrop of global climate change. Most scientists now concur that global heating is leading to more extreme and violent storms. Increasing global temperatures are also associated with the melting of polar ice and therefore increasing likelihood of flooding of coastal lands. Europe, in the summer of 2000, experiences its worst floods in 100 years. In Germany, Austria and the Czech Republic, relentless floodwaters forced thousands of people to evacuate their homes. The year 2005 saw hurricanes Katrina and Rita devastate the Gulf coast region of the US: major oil refineries and pipelines were incapacitated, hundreds killed, hundreds of thousands displaced and a major US city (New Orleans) devastated.

Massive earthquake damage and deaths add to the litany of natural disasters striking the Earth, in addition to the man-made ones. In December 2004 a massive 9.0 earthquake near the Indian Ocean island of Sumatra sparked a wave of deadly tsunamis, causing one of the worst natural disasters in living memory. Approximately 150,000 people died in countries across Asia, and more than 5 million people were left homeless, with Indonesia, Sri Lanka, India and Thailand being the hardest hit. Toward the end of 2005, a massive earthquake hits remote mountainous regions of Pakistan, with a death-toll of 95,000 or more.

Countercultural and Consciousness Expanding Developments

It is not easy to detect any sign of consciousness expansion in this situation or counterculture strength in our present situation. Prior to the invasion of Iraq in 2003, the biggest anti-war protests ever in world history took place – but the US military invaded Iraq anyway. There have been vigorous international protests for more economic justice and fairness at meetings of the WTO and other institutions dedicated to economic globalization – but the WTO, IMF and World Bank continue their neocolonialist policies. Countries of the Southern hemisphere are beginning to create their own trading blocs, making their own agreements and treaties, trying to get out from under the domination by the United States. Nevertheless, the gap between wealthy and poor countries, and classes within countries, continues to widen, and the global economy teeters on the brink of massive collapse.

There have been some historic "firsts" in the global movement toward justice and reconciliation in the first five years of the new millennium: Pope John Paul II offered apologies for sins committed against Jews by the Roman Catholic Church; the South African Truth and Reconciliation Commission walks the difficult path to reconciliation through truth-telling judicial rituals. Former Yugoslav President Milosevic, becomes the first former head of state to face the international war crimes tribunal at The Hague; and former Chilean dictator Pinochet is returned to Chile stripped of immunity and indicted.

Scientific research and theorizing continues to expand the boundaries of the known into the infinite realms of the unknown. In 2003, physicists officially announced the existence of "dark matter," sometimes also referred to as "dark energy," which can only be inferred indirectly, rather than observed. All previously known and observable particles emit or reflect light. However, these observable material particles comprise only 4 percent of the known universe, the remaining 96% being taken up by "dark matter." Space exploration and the search for life on Mars has taken a giant leap forward, when the Mars Odyssey probe found huge reservoirs of ice just beneath the surface, which could indicate conditions suitable for microbial life to develop.

An international consortium of genetic researchers – collectively called the Human Genome Project – announce a scientific breakthrough: they had completely mapped the genetic code of a human chromosome, raising a plethora or medical, legal, and ethical questions, as scientific institutions and medical corporations compete to find profitable applications of the new technologies.

As far as the psychedelic underground culture is concerned, there are small hopeful signs here and there of more official openness to medical and psychiatric research with psychoactive drugs (see:www.maps.org; and www.heffter.org), but there are no indications in mainstream culture or the corporate media that the prohibitionist drug war has abated. It is clear that the underlying purpose of the prohibitionist drug war and the associated disinformation propaganda is similar to the war on terrorism – to instill fear in the population, the mainstream middle class who are too frightened to want to make their own decisions, and want "authorities" to protect them. The climate of fear then facilitates the instillation and maintenance of more "security measures" and imprisonment as a way to generate even more corporate profits and control dissident elements in the population. As journalist William Blum, in his book *Rogue State*, has written:

> Overtly and covertly, legally and illegally, the military-industrial complex has joined forces with the prison-industrial complex, linked further to the omnipresent national security police complex, all clasping hands tightly with the War on Drugs, in a declaration of War on the American people and the Bill of Rights. (Blum, 2000, p. 247).

Perhaps the most significant consciousness expanding development in our time is the *steadily increasing worldwide disclosure about UFO sightings and ET contacts.* Starting in the 1990s, after the collapse of the Soviet Union removed the pretext for cold war secrecy, increasing numbers of ex-military and intelligence whistleblowers, have come forward and added their testimony to that of independent researchers. The emerging consensus from such testimonies and research is two fold: (1) Earth is being visited and observed (*not* invaded) by a number (some say, dozens) of extra-terrestrial civilizations, with diverse agendas, some of which have been around for hundreds, perhaps thousands of years; and (2) ultra-secret groups within the military and intelligence services have conspired to keep knowledge of UFOs and ETs from the public, wanting to use advanced technologies from recovered space-craft and alien contacts for their militaristic domination agendas. As the veils of official government secrecy and disinformation are lifted, the time will come (sooner or later) when there is worldwide conscious public recognition of the presence of scientifically and technologically highly advanced civilizations visiting Earth from other worlds. Recognition of their scientific and technological superiority follows logically from acknowledgement of their presence – from the fact that they are here. While this recognition has already occurred for numerous individuals, when it occurs publicly and openly, it will be, without question, the most significant consciousness expanding event in the history of civilization (Greer, 1999; Mack, 1999; Krapf, 2001; Salla, 2004).

Collapse or New Beginning?

So what is our present situation? With the election of George W. Bush, in the Supreme Court 2000 coup d'état, the launching of pre-emptive wars against nations declared unilaterally to be "terrorist," and his subsequent fraudulent re-election in 2004, the contours of the Imperium Americanum stand ever more nakedly revealed. *It's fascism internally, imperialism externally.* "Fascism" is defined as a dictatorship by oligarchy that merges government, corporate and military leaderships. "Imperialism" is defined as the extension of nationalist hegemony over other nations by military and economic means. This is the explicit, published policy of the present neo-conservative US government, as stated in official documents. "Exporting democracy" and "regime change" have become smoke-screen cover phrases for military intervention to bring about forced subservience to American corporate interests. So-called "free trade" agreements are smoke-screen covers for neo-colonialist exploitation agendas which seek to assure free movements of finance capital, with elimination of any controls in favor of justice for workers or protection of the environment.

In the name of expanding markets and controlling access to key natural resources we've seen the blatant undermining of democratic practice, contempt for international law, restriction of civil liberties and the use of state terrorism to further foreign policy objectives.

We have a dangerously out-of-control rogue state, fascistic and imperialist, arrogantly claiming to lead the world, while ignoring the massive increase in environmental destruction and growing evidence of unprecedented climate change that threatens the survival of civilization. The most heavily armed nation, which is also the chief supplier of arms to all other nations, is engaging in overt and covert military adventures to secure dwindling energy resources. An additional sign of increasing instability is the rising influence on governments of religious fundamentalism – Christian fundamenalists in the US, Jewish fundamentalists in Israel, and Islamic fundamentalists in Arab nations.

The attacks of 9/11 in 2001 obviously delivered a violent external shock to the American and indeed the global economic and political order, as well as collective psyche of Western civilization. In my view, this shock is likely to have even more devastating repercussions, when it is revealed and widely understood, that the attacks not only were used to instill a climate of fear in the American people and justify unlimited aggressive military interventions across the globe, but that they were planned and orchestrated by secret shadow cabals within the US government, for the furtherance of their hegemonic ambitions and control of dwindling global energy resources.[3]

Will these shocks, like the assassinations of progressive leaders in the 1960s, ultimately have the effect of strengthening the culture movements of consciousness transformation? It is true that all of the movements we have identified are still going strong, even stronger than ever, although the trends are more visible and more advanced in other countries, and not the US (or only in certain sub-cultural layers within the US). There is a global movement of resistance to wars of aggression and desire for peace; increasing commitment to racial and ethnic equality; increasing commitment to environmental preservation and conservation; support and protection of equal rights for women and children; acknowledgement of the normality of diversity of sexual orientations; the flourishing of an incredibly rich global culture in the areas of the arts, communications, films, music and lifestyles. We could say also that the heightened knowledge we have of our extra-planetary environment, with space-faring scientific missions, and of our evolutionary cosmology, represents an enormous expansion of collective consciousness.

There is mounting evidence that there may be more astonishing revelations to come from the acknowledged presence of extra-terrestrial visitor civilizations in our planetary environment. If and when this occurs, it will make it possible for the human civilization on Earth to enter consciously into the evolving network of civilizations in our galaxy and beyond. It is my personal belief that such a collective transition will not be possible until we manage to fully establish non-violence as the foundational principle of resolving our differences.

In the high-stakes cosmic game of planetary catastrophe, the Earth has one (or more) trump cards: ecological disasters could occur on such a scale that it would force the diversion of all technological and financial resources to address them. Indeed, mega-disasters stretching national resources are already beginning to happen and likely to elicit further on the ground solidarity among ordinary people everywhere. Of course, it makes no sense to wait or hope for this card to be played.

There may be a general principle at work here that goes something like this: as the oppression and domination of the ruling class in a society or group increases, so do the forces of resistance, revolution and liberation. Growth of the resistance and the counterculture leads in turn to more oppression and domination – "the empire strikes back." Back and forth the movement goes, with three major possible outcomes: *one* is that the oppressive forces gain the upper hand and the subordinate resistance culture is marginalized or wiped out – this is the genocide scenario, exemplified in the story of the indigenous people of the Americas. A *second* possible outcome is that the dominating group is defeated militarily, as with Nazi Germany, or collapses from internal and economic weakness, as with the Soviet Union.

A *third* possible outcome is *synergy* – the different groups or parties find a way to resolve their differences non-violently, the system opens up and responds to feedback, hierarchies of inequality are gradually dismantled, there's a shift in mass consciousness towards economic justice, mutual respect, cooperation and ecological sustainability. The South African movement to end aparthaid is the outstanding example of his scenario in our time.

Those individuals and groups that are more interested in this third alternative outcome, in the preservation of life, human and non-human, in all its astonishing diversity and beauty, than in the enlargement of personal or elite group power and wealth, have the same resources they've always had: the capacity to move into expanded, awakened consciousness; purity and strength of intention and commitment; and the courage and creativity to realize the vision that, in the motto of the tens of thousands who gather annually at World Social Forum meetings, *another world is possible.*

Notes

[1] The political and historical events listed are mostly derived from the time lines listed on the website of the History Channel (www.history.com).

[2] Former French military airtraffic controller Eric Julien has published two books in France on his research on this topic (www.exopoliticsjournal.com).

[3] See the websites: www.911scholars.org; and www.patriotsquestion911.com.

References

Blum, William. *Rogue State*. Monroe, ME: Common Courage Press, 2000.

Corso, Philip J. *The Day After Roswell.* NY: Pocket Books, Simon and Schuster, 1997.

Greer, Steven. *Extraterrestrial Contact – The Evidence and Implications.* Afton, VA: Crossing Point Publications, 1999.

Griffin, David Ray and Scott, Peter Dale (eds). *9/11 and American Empire.* Northampton, MA: Olive Branch Press, Interlink Publishing, 2007.

Grof, Stanislav. *The Psychology of the Future.* Albany, NY: SUNY Press, 2000.

Harner, Michael. *The Way of the Shaman.* San Francisco: Harper & Row, 1980.

Heinberg, Richard. *Power Down.* Gabriola Island, BC, Canada: New Society Publishers, 2004.

Holland, Julie. *Ecstasy: The Complete Guide.* Rochester, VT: Park Street Press, 2001.

Krapf, Phillip. *The Challenge of Contact.* Novato, CA: Origin Press, 2001.

Leary, Tim, Metzner. Ralph and Alpert, Richard. *The Psychedelic Experience.* New Hyde Park, NY: University Books, 1964.

Leary. Timothy. *Flashbacks.* Los Angeles: J. P. Tarcher, 1983.

Mack, John. *Passport to the Cosmos.* NY: Crown Publishers, 1999.

Markoff, John. *What the Dormouse Said.* NY: Penguin Viking, 2005.

Metzner, Ralph. *Green Psychology.* Rochester, VT: Inner Traditions

International, 1999.

Metzner, Ralph (ed.) *Sacred Mushroom of Visions – Teonanácatl.* Rochester, VT: Park Street Press, 2005.

Metzner, Ralph (ed.) *Sacred Vine of Spirits – Ayahuasca.* Rochester, VT: Park Street Press, 2006.

Ruppert, Michael. *Crossing the Rubicon.* Gabriola Island, BC, Canada: New Society Publishers, 2004.

Salla, Michael. *Exopolitics – The pratical implications of extraterrestrial presence.* Tempe, AZ: Dandelion Press, 2004.

Scott, Peter Dale. *Drugs, Oil and War.* Lanham, MD: Rowan & Littlefield Publishers, 2003.

Tarnas, Richard. *Cosmos and Psyche.* NY: Viking, 2006.

Green Earth Foundation

Harmonizing Humanity with Earth and Spirit

The Green Earth Foundation is an educational and research organization dedicated to the healing and harmonizing of the relationships between humanity and the Earth, through a recognition of the energetic and spiritual interconnectedness of all life-forms in all worlds. Our strategic objectives are to help bring about changes in attitudes, values, perceptions, and worldviews that are based on ecological balance and respect for the integrity of all life. Our areas of research interest include consciousness studies, shamanism and Earth mythology, and green and eco-psychology. Green Earth Foundation also sponsors the *Metzner Alchemical Divination®* training program.

Green Earth Founation
is producing and co-publishing a new series of books
by Ralph Metzner, Ph.D. –

THE ECOLOGY OF CONSCIOUSNESS

1. The Expansion of Consciousness
2. The Predicament of Domination
3. Varieties of States of Consciousness
4. Alchemical Divination
5. The Psychology of Incarnation, Birth and Death
6. Worlds Within and Worlds Beyond

The Green Earth Foundation is a 501 (c) (3) non-profit, educational and research organization. Address: P.O. Box 327, El Verano. CA 95433. Internet: www.greenearthfound.org

Alchemical Divination

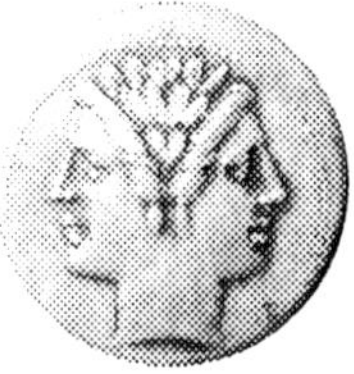

Alchemy is the ancient art and science of elemental transformation. The focus of alchemical practicioners was healing and what we would nowadays call psychotherapy, as well as spiritual growth and understanding. *Alchemy*, like shamanism and yoga, with which it is related, involves teachings and practices of physical, psychic and spiritual transformation, expressed in the imaginal language of material transformation.

Divination is the practice of seeking healing, insight and guidance from inner sources commonly called the "spirit world" or "divine world", or one's intuition or Higher Self. We are most familiar with divination accessories or tools such as the Tarot, the I Ching, or the Nordic Runes; but the essence of the process is the asking of questions and receiving answers from inner sources of knowledge and guidance.

The *alchemical divinations* developed by Ralph Metzner are processes of structured intuitive inquiry, using light-fire yoga methods for a heightened state of concentrative awareness. We work in the spirit of the Roman deity Janus, god of doorways, passages and transitions, whose two faces look in a balanced way into the past and the future.

The basic purpose of these alchemical divinations is to help individuals obtain deeper experiential understanding, problem resolution and visionary inspiration for their life path in its intrapsychic, interpersonal, professional, creative and spiritual dimensions.

The *Metzner Alchemical Divination®* training program consists of three, modular 5-day workshops, taught in the US and in Europe, in which one learns the divinations for oneself, and how to conduct them for others.

Please consult the website: www.metzneralchemicaldivination.org, for details.